All

you have to know

about

The Urology

Caregiver

MARTIN STERLING

Table of contents

Chapter 1: Introduction to the role of the nursing auxiliary in urology   15

- **The caregiver's main missions**   16

  ○ Accompanying the patient in hospital   16

  ○ Collaboration with the multidisciplinary team   17

  ○ Basic care and comfort management   19

- **Specific features of the urology department**   21

  ○ Presentation of common pathologies (urinary tract infections, prostate cancer, urinary lithiasis, etc.).   21

  ○ Difference between urology, surgery, oncology and palliative care services   23

- **The caregiver's essential role in the care process**   26

  ○ The importance of listening and empathy   26

  ○ Interface between patient and medical team   27

Chapter 2: Anatomy and urological pathologies   31

- **Basic anatomy**   32

  ◦ Male and female urinary tract   32

  ◦ Functional anatomy: kidneys, bladder, urethra, prostate   34

- **Common pathologies**   36

  ◦ Prostate cancer, bladder cancer, kidney failure   36

  ◦ Urinary tract infections: cystitis, pyelonephritis   38

  ◦ Urinary incontinence: causes and consequences   40

- **Urological treatments and procedures**   42

  ◦ Medical and surgical treatments   42

  ◦ Different types of catheter (ureteral, suprapubic, etc.)   44

  ◦ Lithotripsy, prostatectomy, nephrectomy, cystoscopy   47

Chapter 3: Daily management of the urology patient   51

- **The key role of hygiene and asepsis**   52

◦ Preventing nosocomial infections 52

◦ Sterile care techniques (probes, catheters) 54

◦ Hand washing and equipment preparation 56

• **Basic and technical care** 58

◦ Intimate hygiene and specific hygiene care 58

◦ Monitoring drains and probes 61

◦ Post-operative care: scar monitoring, pain management 63

• **Patient comfort and mobility** 66

◦ Mobilization assistance after surgery 66

◦ Pressure sore prevention and skin monitoring 68

◦ Patient set-up for examinations and procedures (cystoscopy, radiology) 71

Chapter 4: Emergency management in urology

75

• **Recognizing and responding to urological complications** 76

◦ Acute urinary retention 76

○   Severe urinary tract infection: urological sepsis   78

○   Post-operative bleeding   81

• **The caregiver's role in the emergency team**   83

○   Managing stress and emotions in emergency situations   83

○   Collaborate effectively with the medical team   86

○   Manage logistics (emergency room preparation, close monitoring)   89

• **Precautions and protocol in the event of a crisis**   92

○   Ensuring patient safety   92

○   Protocol in the event of severe infection or postoperative complications   95

Chapter 5: The patient-caregiver relationship in urology   99

• **Psychological support for patients**   100

○   Anxiety about urological surgery   100

○   Psychological impact of pathologies such as incontinence or cancer   102

◦ The importance of non-verbal communication   105

• **Helping patients accept their illness**   108

     ◦ The caregiver's role in patient information   108

     ◦ Respecting privacy and modesty during care   111

     ◦ End-of-life support in urological palliative care   114

• **Managing relationships with loved ones**   117

     ◦ Involving family members in daily care   117

     ◦ Appropriate communication with the family   120

Chapter 6: Technological tools and innovations in urology   123

• **Cutting-edge diagnostic and treatment technologies**   124

     ◦ CT scan, MRI, urological ultrasound   124

     ◦ Surgical robotics and minimally invasive procedures   127

• **The impact of new technologies on the caregiver's work**   130

    ◦   Management of technological   130
           equipment (probes, monitoring
           devices)

    ◦   Assist the surgical team in the use   133
           of robots

• Ongoing training and adaptation to   136
innovation

    ◦   Importance of continuing   136
           education

    ◦   Participate in training sessions on   139
           new technologies

Chapter 7: Ethical issues in urology care   143

• Respect the patient's dignity in all   144
circumstances

    ◦   Managing delicate situations   144
           during intimate care

    ◦   Ensuring the confidentiality of   147
           medical data

    ◦   Adapting one's behavior to the   149
           patient's beliefs and values

• Ethical dilemmas specific to urology   153

    ◦   Informed consent for invasive   153
           procedures

◦ End-of-life and palliative care issues   156

◦ Handling requests from patients who disagree with medical practices   158

• **The ethics of new technologies in urology**   162

◦ The impact of robots and artificial intelligence on the caregiver-patient relationship   162

◦ The ethics of genetic sequencing and sensitive data   164

Chapter 8: Rare and complex pathologies in urology   169

• **Rare urological diseases: a challenge for caregivers**   170

◦ Caring for patients with rare diseases   170

◦ Adapting care and protocols for specific cases   172

• **Complex pathologies and co-morbidities**   175

◦ Managing patients with multiple chronic conditions (diabetes, hypertension, etc.)   175

◦ Care for frail, elderly patients   179

- **The role of the caregiver in clinical trials**   182

   ◦ Participate in the follow-up of patients included in research protocols   182

   ◦ Medication management and specific care for patients in clinical research   185

Chapter 9: Therapeutic patient education in urology   189

- **The caregiver's role in patient education**   190

   ◦ Explain care and treatment to patients and their families   190

   ◦ Information on healthy living after surgery   193

- **Helping patients to manage their own health**   196

   ◦ Help understand ongoing care (home catheterization, catheters, etc.)   196

   ◦ Provide post-operative follow-up: manage appointments, monitor recovery   198

- **Collaboration with nurses and doctors for therapeutic education**   202

◦ Organize patient information sessions	202
◦ Adapt speech to patients' level of understanding	205

Conclusion: The future of the urology orderly — 209

- **Future challenges for urology care** — 210
  - ◦ An aging population and an increase in urological pathologies — 210
  - ◦ Developments in care techniques and robotization — 212
- **The growing role of the caregiver in a changing medical context** — 216
  - ◦ Towards greater responsibility in care — 216
  - ◦ Helping patients to manage their own health — 219
- **Training to progress in the nursing auxiliary profession** — 221
  - ◦ Access to specializations — 221
  - ◦ Career prospects in the urology department — 224

« *In urology, it's simple: when it flows, it's a good sign... except when it shouldn't!* »

Chapter 1

Introduction to the role of the nursing auxiliary in urology

The caregiver's main missions
      ◦   Accompanying the patient in hospital
Accompanying patients in the hospital environment, particularly in a urology department, is a fundamental aspect of the nursing auxiliary's role. It's not simply a question of providing technical care, but of offering comprehensive, human care, adapted to the individual needs of each patient. The caregiver is often the first person with whom the patient comes into contact, and plays a key role throughout the patient's stay. This relationship begins on admission and continues right through to the patient's discharge, creating a bond of trust that is essential to quality care.

In urology, patients can find themselves in situations of physical or psychological discomfort, as the pathologies linked to this specialty often affect intimate and sensitive areas. Shyness, embarrassment and sometimes anxiety are frequent emotions that caregivers must learn to recognize and soothe. By listening attentively and communicating appropriately, the caregiver helps to reduce the patient's apprehension about treatments or procedures.

Support begins at the reception desk, where the orderly takes the time to explain the procedures, orient the patient in the hospital, and make sure he or she understands what's going to happen. This initial phase is essential to reduce anxiety, particularly in a department like urology, where examinations (cystoscopy, urinary catheterization) and procedures can be experienced as intrusive. The caregiver's benevolent, reassuring attitude becomes the patient's reference point.

Throughout the hospital stay, the nursing auxiliary is responsible for creating an environment conducive to healing, both physically and emotionally. He/she ensures that basic needs are met: hygiene, comfort, nutrition, while taking into account the specifics of the patient's urological condition. For example, for a patient who has undergone prostate surgery, the caregiver will need to pay particular attention to the management of urinary drainage, while explaining to the patient the steps involved in his recovery. Patients must understand that their recovery depends in part on their active participation in care, and the caregiver is there to encourage them, inform them and answer any questions they may have.

Caregivers also play an essential role in providing psychological support for patients. In urology, certain conditions such as incontinence or erectile dysfunction can affect self-esteem and quality of life. The caregiver's active listening and discretion enable patients to express themselves freely, without judgment. This relationship of trust is essential, as it promotes greater adherence to care and better collaboration between patient and medical staff.

Finally, support does not end when the patient leaves hospital. The caregiver prepares the patient for his or her return home, ensuring that the patient understands the post-hospitalization instructions: how to manage care at home, how to use specific equipment (urinary catheters, drainage bags), and the warning signs that should prompt consultation. The caregiver thus becomes a pillar not only of medical care, but also of the patient's general well-being throughout the hospital stay.

This holistic approach, based on listening, closeness and respect, makes the nursing auxiliary an indispensable player in urological care, helping to humanize care in a technical environment that is sometimes perceived as cold.

     ○   Collaboration with the multidisciplinary team
Collaboration with the multidisciplinary team is one of the cornerstones of the urology orderly's work. The urology department is a complex environment, where patients often require varied, technical and personalized care, involving numerous healthcare professionals. The nursing auxiliary plays an essential role in ensuring the smooth flow of care, by integrating fully into this team, and ensuring effective coordination between the various members. This collaboration

goes far beyond the simple execution of tasks, and involves genuine communication, constant adaptation to the patient's needs and anticipation of future actions.

The multidisciplinary urology team generally includes urologists, surgeons, nurses, physiotherapists, anesthetists, psychologists, and sometimes oncologists, depending on the pathologies treated. Each professional contributes his or her specific expertise to ensure comprehensive patient care. The nursing auxiliary, although often perceived as an operator, is in fact a central player in this dynamic. They act as a link between the various parties involved, working closely with the patient on a day-to-day basis, and observing changes in his or her condition.

Communication is one of the key aspects of this collaboration. The caregiver conveys essential information about the patient's physical and emotional state. For example, if a patient shows signs of discomfort, a post-operative complication, or a change in behavior, the caregiver immediately informs the nurse or doctor in charge, enabling rapid and appropriate intervention. This early warning role is crucial, as the caregiver is often the one who spends the most time at the patient's bedside, and can spot subtle signs of deterioration before they become critical.

In addition, the nursing auxiliary works closely with the nurses in the execution of technical care. In urology, this includes tasks such as managing urinary catheters, monitoring drains, and assisting with certain medical procedures. The nursing auxiliary must not only master these gestures, but also know how to adapt to the specific needs of the patient, according to the instructions given by the medical team. Good collaboration therefore relies on mutual trust, respect for each other's skills, and clear, regular communication.

During surgery, the orderly also plays an indirect role in preparing the patient, ensuring that pre-operative protocols are followed (antiseptic cleansing, administration of prescribed medication), and looking after the patient's emotional well-being before the operation. After the operation, they play an active role in post-operative monitoring, assisting the nurse with pain management, monitoring vital signs, and early mobilization of the patient. The nursing auxiliary becomes an indispensable link between the operating room, the ward nurses and the patient.

Collaboration with physiotherapists is also frequent in the urology department, particularly for patients who have undergone operations affecting mobility or requiring pelvic floor re-education. The nursing auxiliary often prepares patients for physiotherapy sessions, helps them to settle in, and ensures that they are in the best possible condition to follow their treatment. They also play an important role in monitoring patient progress and communicating this information to the physiotherapists.

In addition to physical care, the multidisciplinary urology team also includes mental health professionals such as psychologists and psychiatrists. Certain urological conditions, such as incontinence disorders or prostate cancer, can have a considerable emotional impact on patients. Through their regular contact with patients, nursing auxiliaries are often on the front line in spotting signs of psychological distress. In collaboration with psychologists, they can help identify emotional support needs and implement strategies to improve the patient's well-being.

○   Basic care and comfort management

The management of basic care and comfort is an essential component of the work of the urology care assistant, as it forms the very basis of day-to-day patient care. In this department, care is not limited to technical medical procedures or surgical interventions, but encompasses all gestures aimed at ensuring patients' well-being, dignity and comfort. This care is essential for maintaining a good quality of life, preventing complications and promoting recovery, particularly for hospitalized or post-operative patients.

The caregiver begins each day with an assessment of each patient's basic needs. These needs include personal hygiene, nutrition, physical comfort and maintaining mobility. In urology, hygiene is of paramount importance, as the pathologies treated directly affect the urinary tract, an area sensitive to infection. The nursing auxiliary therefore takes charge of patient grooming, ensuring compliance with asepsis protocols, particularly for patients with urinary catheters or drains. Careful grooming not only helps to prevent infections, but also ensures the patient's physical comfort, by making them feel clean and comfortable.

In the context of hygiene, the nursing auxiliary is also responsible for intimate care, such as changing incontinence pads or maintaining catheters. This type of care requires great delicacy, as it touches on the patient's dignity. The caregiver must show respect, listening skills and empathy to put the patient at ease, while maintaining a high level of technical skill to avoid any complications. Discretion and professionalism are essential in these intimate moments, when the caregiver-patient relationship is based on mutual trust.

Patient comfort is not limited to personal hygiene. The caregiver must also ensure that the patient is comfortable in bed or in the chair, by adjusting cushions, ensuring correct body position to prevent bedsores, and facilitating regular changes of position. In urology, certain procedures, such as prostatectomy or kidney surgery, can entail prolonged periods of immobilization. It is therefore crucial to maintain constant vigilance over the skin, to ensure gentle mobilization of the limbs, and to prevent complications linked to bed rest, such as bedsores or thrombosis.

The nursing auxiliary also plays a vital role in pain management and post-operative comfort. He or she may be required to monitor the patient's pain, adapt the environment to the patient's needs (light, temperature, bed position) and collaborate with the nurse in the management of analgesics. Comfort is a key aspect of convalescence, and a patient who feels comfortable in his or her environment heals more quickly.

Nutrition is another area in which the nursing auxiliary is fully involved. Depending on medical prescriptions, he or she may be responsible for distributing meals, but also for helping patients who have difficulty feeding themselves, particularly after surgery or in cases of physical weakness. Good nutrition is essential to recovery, and the caregiver ensures that the patient is well hydrated and nourished, while respecting specific diets (salt-free diet, water diet, etc.) prescribed for urological pathologies.

In addition to physical care, the caregiver must be attentive to the patient's psychological comfort. A patient who feels well cared for, listened to and respected has a better hospital stay. Through their daily presence, caregivers are often the people to whom patients confide, sharing their fears and doubts. They can play a calming role by answering questions, explaining care and providing a reassuring presence, especially at difficult moments such as before surgery or in situations of intense pain.

Managing basic care and comfort is not just about meeting immediate needs. It also involves anticipating the patient's future needs. This may involve careful monitoring of the patient's general condition, ongoing assessment of his or her needs in terms of hygiene, mobility and nutrition, as well as constant communication with the nursing team to adapt care as necessary. This anticipation helps to avoid complications, maintain a high level of comfort, and ensure that the patient can live his or her hospitalization as serenely as possible.

Specific features of the urology department
- Presentation of common pathologies (urinary tract infections, prostate cancer, urinary lithiasis, etc.).

The presentation of common pathologies in urology is a crucial step in understanding the diversity of conditions that nursing auxiliaries are likely to encounter in their day-to-day work. The Urology Department treats a wide range of conditions, from benign infections to serious cancers, as well as functional disorders of the urinary tract. The three main disease categories are urinary tract infections, prostate cancer and urinary lithiasis, each with its own specific management and care requirements.

Urinary tract infections are among the most frequent pathologies in urology, affecting both men and women, although the latter are often more affected. They result from the proliferation of bacteria in the urinary system, and can manifest themselves at different levels: from the bladder (cystitis) to the kidneys (pyelonephritis). Typical symptoms include pain on urination (burning), frequent urination, and sometimes lower back pain, as well as fever in the case of kidney infection. For the caregiver, managing urinary tract infections involves careful monitoring of the patient's condition, in particular by checking the urine (presence of blood, abnormal coloration) and ensuring that the patient follows prescribed hydration and antibiotic treatment instructions. Rigorous hygiene is essential to prevent recurrences, especially in patients with urinary catheters, who are more exposed to these infections.

Another major area of urology concerns **cancers**, and more specifically **prostate cancer**, which is one of the most frequently diagnosed cancers in men, particularly after the age of 50. The prostate, a small gland located beneath the bladder, can develop cancerous tumors which, if not detected and treated in time, can spread to the rest of the body. Symptoms of prostate cancer may be discreet in the early stages, but as the disease progresses, they include difficulty in urinating, a feeling of not emptying the bladder completely, and sometimes pain in the lower back or pelvis. Screening is often based on a prostate-specific antigen (PSA) test and a digital rectal examination, followed by a biopsy to confirm the diagnosis. The role of the caregiver in caring for prostate cancer patients is vital, both physically and emotionally. They accompany the patient through all stages of treatment, whether surgery (prostatectomy), radiotherapy or chemotherapy, providing rigorous post-operative follow-up and ensuring that the patient retains maximum comfort and dignity. Listening and empathy are crucial here, as the diagnosis of cancer can lead to deep-seated anxieties linked to the disease itself, but also to treatments that can have repercussions on quality of life (incontinence, erectile dysfunction).

Urinary lithiasis, also known as kidney stones, is another frequent pathology in the urology department. Stones are hard crystals that form in the kidneys or bladder, and can cause intense pain when they block the urinary tract. The pain, often described as one of the most severe by patients, is localized in the lower back and may radiate to the abdomen or groin. It is often accompanied by nausea and vomiting. There are many causes of stones: insufficient hydration, a diet rich in salt or protein, and a family history. The treatment of stones can range from the administration of medication to facilitate their expulsion, to more invasive procedures such as extracorporeal lithotripsy, which consists of fragmenting the stones using shock waves, or surgery in more severe cases. Caregivers play a key role in monitoring patients with lithiasis, making sure they are properly hydrated, helping them to manage pain, and overseeing stone expulsion, often a dreaded but necessary moment for recovery.

In addition to these major pathologies, urology also treats other common conditions such as **urinary incontinence**, which can be linked to age, trauma or certain surgical procedures, as well as functional disorders such as **dysuria** (difficulty in urinating) and **benign prostatic hyperplasia** (enlargement of the prostate gland without being cancerous). These conditions, although often perceived as benign, can have a considerable impact on patients' quality of life, requiring special attention from caregivers.

        ◦   Difference between urology, surgery, oncology and
             palliative care services
The difference between urology, surgery, oncology and palliative care departments is essential to understanding the patient's care pathway and the specific role played by the caregiver in each of these environments. Each of these services has its own

particularities, modes of operation and types of care, but they are often complementary in the treatment of patients with urological pathologies.

The **Urology Department** specializes in the diagnosis and treatment of disorders of the urinary and male genital systems. The department deals with a wide range of pathologies, including urinary tract infections, kidney stones, incontinence, as well as prostate, bladder and kidney cancers. Urology combines medical and surgical treatments, and patients are cared for in consultations, light procedures (such as cystoscopy) or hospitalizations for more complex care. The urology orderly is at the heart of day-to-day care management: ensuring patient comfort, monitoring medical devices (catheters, drains) and playing an active role in infection prevention, a key issue in this department. In urology, a close relationship with patients is essential, as they may be confronted with pathologies that affect intimate areas, requiring great sensitivity and a profound respect for modesty.

The **surgery department** focuses on surgical interventions that may be required for urological diseases, but also in many other medical fields. In urology, surgery is used to treat pathologies such as prostate cancer and kidney tumors, or to remove urinary calculi that are refractory to drug treatment. Patients are referred to this department for procedures that can be major, such as radical prostatectomy, or less invasive, such as shock wave lithotripsy. In this context, the nursing auxiliary helps prepare the patient before the operation (pre-operative hygiene, stress management), and then ensures close post-operative monitoring. Pain management, early mobilization and scar monitoring are also part of their duties. The surgical department is therefore an environment where constant vigilance is required, as patients may experience post-operative complications, and rapid intervention in the event of a problem is crucial.

The **oncology department** is more specifically dedicated to the treatment of cancers, including urological cancers such as those of the prostate, bladder or kidney. Unlike the surgery department, oncology focuses primarily on treatment by chemotherapy, radiotherapy or immunotherapy, aimed at destroying cancer cells. Oncology patients may be followed over the long term, and the caregiver plays an essential role in supporting them. Oncology treatments are often heavy and exhausting, with significant side-effects such as fatigue, nausea, pain and low morale. Caregivers not only ensure patients' physical comfort, they also provide psychological support. They act as a point of reference on an often long and difficult journey, helping patients to overcome moments of discouragement. Oncology is a department where the human dimension and empathy are particularly important, as patients undergo ordeals that are not only physical, but also emotional.

Finally, **palliative care** is a service dedicated to patients in the terminal phase of their illness, when curative treatments are no longer effective and the aim becomes pain relief and improved quality of life. In urology, patients with advanced cancers, notably of the prostate or bladder, may be transferred to palliative care if the disease progresses despite treatment. The role of the caregiver in this department is above all to ensure patients' comfort and to accompany them with dignity to the end of their lives. This involves comprehensive care: pain management, psychological support, comfort care (grooming, feeding), as well as an attentive, caring presence. The palliative care assistant must also be able to support relatives, who are often very present in this department, by informing them and accompanying them through this difficult stage. Here, more than in any other department, the human dimension takes precedence over the technical, and the caregiver must demonstrate great compassion and absolute respect for the patient's wishes and needs.

The caregiver's essential role in the care process
            ◦   The importance of listening and empathy

The importance of listening and empathy in the caregiver's work, particularly in a department as sensitive as urology, cannot be overestimated. These qualities are at the heart of efficient, humane and respectful patient care. Urology deals with pathologies that often touch on the intimacy and dignity of individuals. In this context, listening and empathy help create a bond of trust between caregiver and patient, reduce anxiety and improve patient compliance.

Listening, in this context, is not limited to hearing the patient's words. It involves active attention to what the patient is expressing, whether verbally or through body language. Many patients are reluctant to share some of their concerns, particularly when it comes to intimate problems such as incontinence, erectile dysfunction or pain during urination. The caregiver must therefore be able to decode non-verbal signs - discomfort in posture, a fleeting glance, an expression of discomfort - so as to be able to broach these delicate subjects without forcing the conversation, but leaving the patient the necessary space to express himself. This ability to detect subtle signs of concern or discomfort is often crucial to the patient's well-being.

Empathy, on the other hand, goes beyond a simple intellectual understanding of the patient's suffering. It's the ability to put oneself in the other person's shoes, to feel what they're going through, and to adapt one's behavior accordingly. In urology, where patients may feel ashamed or frustrated by their illness, empathy enables the caregiver to create an environment where the patient feels respected and understood, even in moments of great vulnerability. For example, when a patient has to be probed or undergo intrusive examinations, the way the caregiver approaches these moments, with gentleness and empathy, can transform a stressful experience into a more bearable, even reassuring interaction.

A patient who feels listened to and taken into consideration, not only in his or her physical needs but also in his or her emotions, is more likely to cooperate and accept the care offered. Empathy also enables caregivers to tailor their care to the specific needs and emotions of each patient. For example, a patient faced with a prostate cancer diagnosis might express fears not only for his immediate health, but also for the impact of the disease on his personal and intimate life. By taking the time to listen to these concerns and responding empathetically, the caregiver offers essential emotional support that helps the patient to better manage his or her situation.

Listening and empathy are also essential in managing relationships with families. Patients' loved ones can also be upset, worried and sometimes frustrated by the situation. By listening to their concerns and showing empathy, caregivers can help ease tensions and clarify misunderstandings. Accompanying families, particularly in end-of-life or critical illness situations, is a key component of care. Families, like patients, need to feel that they are being heard and that their feelings are being taken into account. A kind word, a gesture of encouragement or simply an attentive ear can make a significant difference to these loved ones, who often feel powerless in the face of illness.

Empathy also enables caregivers to manage emotionally difficult situations. In urology, certain operations or treatments can have after-effects that profoundly affect a patient's self-image. A man suffering from incontinence after surgery, or having lost certain erectile functions, may feel profound distress. By showing empathy, the caregiver can help these patients not to feel reduced to their symptoms or illness, but to see themselves as individuals with complex emotions and needs.

◦ Interface between patient and medical team

The nursing auxiliary plays a key role as the interface between the patient and the medical team. This role is often invisible, but fundamental, as it ensures fluid and efficient communication, while guaranteeing that the patient's needs are correctly relayed to healthcare professionals. This intermediary position requires not only technical mastery of care, but also great listening, observation and communication skills.

Patients, especially in a department like urology, where pathologies touch on intimacy and dignity, may be reluctant to express their concerns or discomforts directly to a doctor or nurse. The caregiver's daily proximity to the patient often makes him or her the first person to confide in. Whether it's about troublesome symptoms, pain, concerns about a treatment or simply a need for more information, the patient often finds an attentive ear in the caregiver. This bond of trust that develops enables the caregiver to capture valuable information that might otherwise escape the medical team. The caregiver's role is to convey this information clearly and precisely, so that the doctor or nurse can adapt the patient's care accordingly.

Transmitting information requires a high degree of rigor. The caregiver must be able to describe the patient's condition objectively: evolution of clinical signs, observation of changes in behavior, reactions to treatments or interventions, etc. These observations, although seemingly anecdotal at first glance, are often decisive in adjusting treatment. These observations, although seemingly anecdotal at first glance, are often decisive in adjusting treatment. For example, a patient who suddenly becomes quieter or irritable could be hiding pain or discomfort. If the caregiver picks up this information and passes it on to the nurse or doctor, it may lead to a reassessment of pain management, or to further tests to detect a complication. It's this constant vigilance, combined with the ability to communicate, that makes the caregiver a key player in medical care.

In the other direction, the caregiver is also responsible for passing on instructions from the medical team to the patient. This may include instructions on post-operative care, management of medical devices (such as urinary catheters), or recommendations for recovery at home. The caregiver must ensure that the patient has understood these instructions, re-explain them if necessary and, above all, adapt them to the patient's language. This is crucial, as medical information can sometimes be complex or overly technical. The caregiver's close relationship with the patient enables him or her to personalize the message, so that the patient feels confident and clearly understands what is expected of him or her.

This interface role is also expressed in the patient's emotional response to medical decisions. When a doctor announces a difficult diagnosis or prescribes a complex treatment, the patient may feel overwhelmed or anxious. As a trusted interlocutor, the caregiver can play a mediating role. He or she is often the one who gathers the patient's initial reactions, doubts, fears and misunderstandings. By listening carefully to these emotions, the caregiver is able to pass on these questions to the doctors or nurses, while reassuring the patient and helping him or her to better understand the situation. This constant dialogue between patient and medical team, facilitated by the caregiver, ensures that the patient never feels abandoned or ignored in his or her care journey.

The role of interface also takes on its full meaning in the coordination of care. The nursing auxiliary works closely with all healthcare professionals, whether nurses, doctors, physiotherapists or specialists. When a patient needs to move from one department to another (for example, from urology to surgery for an operation), the orderly ensures that important information about the patient's condition is passed on correctly, and that continuity of care is guaranteed. They also ensure that the patient is physically and mentally prepared for each step, understands what is going to happen, and is optimally cared for.

Chapter 2

Anatomy and urological pathologies

Basic anatomy

◦ Male and female urinary tract

The urinary tract, in both men and women, plays a fundamental role in eliminating waste from the body, filtering blood and excreting toxins in the form of urine. Although the structure and function of this apparatus are broadly similar in both sexes, there are anatomical differences that influence the way certain pathologies manifest themselves and are managed. Understanding these differences is essential for appropriate patient management, particularly in urological care.

The male urinary system comprises the kidneys, ureters, bladder and urethra. The **kidneys** are two bean-shaped organs located on either side of the spine, whose main function is to filter blood to eliminate waste and excess water, forming urine. This urine is then transported to the **bladder** via the **ureters**, two fine ducts that connect the kidneys to the bladder. The bladder is a muscular organ that acts as a reservoir for urine until it is evacuated.

In men, the urethra, which carries urine from the bladder to the outside of the body, passes through the **prostate**, a walnut-sized gland located beneath the bladder. This structure is unique to male anatomy and plays a key role in the reproductive system, contributing to sperm formation. However, the prostate is also a common site of pathologies, including prostate cancer and benign prostatic hypertrophy, a non-cancerous increase in the volume of this gland that can lead to urinary problems such as difficulty urinating or a frequent urge to go to the toilet. As men age, they are often confronted with prostate-related urinary disorders, making this gland central to male urological management.

The male urethra, which is longer than the female urethra, has a dual function: not only does it allow the evacuation of urine, but also the passage of sperm during ejaculation. This anatomical peculiarity explains why certain pathologies, such as urinary tract infections, are less frequent in men, but can be more serious when they do occur, as bacteria have to travel a longer path to reach the bladder.

The **female urinary tract** also comprises the kidneys, ureters, bladder and urethra, but with some notable anatomical differences. The **kidneys** and **ureters** function in the same way as in men, filtering blood and transporting urine to the bladder. However, the **female bladder** is closer to the internal reproductive organs, notably the uterus and ovaries, which can sometimes complicate the management of urological pathologies in women, particularly during pregnancy or the menopause.

The main difference between the male and female urinary systems lies in the **urethra**. In women, the urethra is much shorter than in men, measuring around 4 cm, compared with 15 to 20 cm in men. This anatomical peculiarity makes women more vulnerable to **urinary tract infections**, as bacteria have more direct access to the bladder. Indeed, the female urethra is located close to the anus, facilitating the migration of germs to the urinary tract. This is why cystitis, or bladder infections, are much more common in women, particularly after sexual intercourse or during the menopause, when estrogen production declines, leading to changes in the urethral mucosa.

Unlike the male urethra, the female urethra has no reproductive function. However, because of its proximity to the reproductive organs, urinary disorders can sometimes occur in women in connection with gynecological pathologies, such as prolapses (organ descent), which often occur after childbirth or due to weakening of the pelvic floor. These prolapses can lead to urinary difficulties or leakage, and require specific management by urological and gynecological teams.

Thus, the anatomy of the male and female urinary tract, although similar in its main functions, presents differences that influence the development and management of pathologies. In men, the prostate plays a central role in age-related urinary disorders, while in women, the proximity of the urethra to the anus and its short length explain the higher frequency of urinary tract infections. These anatomical differences must be taken into account by the caregiver in managing daily care and preventing complications. A good knowledge of this anatomy enables care to be adapted to each patient, the underlying causes of their disorders to be understood, and personalized, effective support to be provided for both men and women.

      ◦   Functional anatomy: kidneys, bladder, urethra, prostate

The functional anatomy of the kidneys, bladder, urethra and prostate form a system essential to the filtration and evacuation of the body's waste products, while also playing a role in water and electrolyte balance. Although interconnected, these organs each perform specific functions which, together, ensure the proper functioning of the urinary tract, and, in the case of the prostate, an important contribution to the male reproductive system.

The **kidneys** are the main organs of the urinary system. Located on either side of the spinal column, just below the rib cage, their main function is to filter the blood to remove metabolic waste and maintain the balance of water, mineral salts and electrolytes. Every day, the kidneys filter around 180 liters of blood plasma, but only 1 to 2 liters of urine are produced. This urine is made up of water, salts, urea and other substances that the body must eliminate. The kidneys also perform other vital functions: they regulate blood pressure, produce hormones (such as erythropoietin, which stimulates the production of red blood cells), and contribute to the body's acid-base balance. The filtration process in the kidneys takes place in microscopic units called **nephrons**, which filter the blood and separate substances to be eliminated from those to be reabsorbed. The waste products thus collected are transformed into urine, which is then evacuated via the **ureters**, fine ducts connecting the kidneys to the bladder.

The **bladder**, located in the lower abdomen, acts as a reservoir for urine. Its muscular wall, composed of the detrusor muscle, is capable of relaxing to store up to 500 ml of urine, but it can also contract to expel urine during micturition. The functioning of the bladder is controlled by a complex nervous system that activates

34

contractions when the bladder is full, and coordinates the opening of the urethral sphincter to allow the evacuation of urine. The caregiver needs to understand bladder physiology to monitor urinary disorders common in certain clinical contexts, such as urinary retention, incontinence or infection. Urinary catheterization, frequently used in urology, requires particular attention to hygiene and infection prevention to avoid complications.

The urethra, the tube that connects the bladder to the outside of the body, has a different structure in men and women. In men, it measures between 15 and 20 cm and passes through the prostate before entering the penis. The urethra plays a dual role: it enables the evacuation of urine, but also the passage of sperm during ejaculation. In women, the urethra is much shorter, around 4 cm, and lies just above the vaginal opening. This shorter anatomy in women makes them more susceptible to urinary tract infections, as bacteria have a shorter route to travel to reach the bladder. Monitoring for infections, irritation or urethral dysfunction is essential to prevent more serious complications, such as kidney infections.

Finally, in men, the **prostate** is a specific gland that surrounds the urethra at the outlet of the bladder. It plays an important role in the reproductive system, producing part of the seminal fluid that nourishes and transports sperm. As it ages, however, the prostate can become problematic. **Benign prostatic hyperplasia** (BPH), a non-cancerous enlargement of the prostate gland, is common in men over the age of 50, and can cause difficulty in urination by compressing the urethra. Symptoms include a frequent urge to urinate, difficulty in starting urination, or a feeling of not emptying the bladder completely. **Prostate cancer**, another common problem, can also cause similar symptoms but requires a much more complex treatment, often including surgery, radiotherapy or hormone therapy. Monitoring prostate function is therefore essential in middle-aged men.

Taken as a whole, these organs work in close collaboration to ensure efficient elimination of bodily waste while maintaining a vital internal balance. The kidneys filter blood, the bladder stores urine, the urethra evacuates it, and in men, the prostate is also involved in reproductive function. Each organ has specific vulnerabilities, and a thorough knowledge of their functional anatomy enables the caregiver to monitor for signs of dysfunction, actively participate in care and ensure appropriate management of pathologies linked to this complex apparatus.

Common pathologies
  ◦　　Prostate cancer, bladder cancer, kidney failure
Prostate cancer, **bladder cancer** and **renal failure** are three of the main serious pathologies encountered in urology, each with different characteristics, treatments and impacts on patients. Although they affect distinct organs of the urinary tract, they share common challenges in terms of early diagnosis, therapeutic management and support for patients, both physically and emotionally.

Prostate cancer is one of the most common cancers in men, particularly after the age of 50. The prostate, a gland located below the bladder, plays a key role in reproduction by producing part of the seminal fluid, but it is also a vulnerable site for tumor formation. The majority of prostate cancers develop slowly and often cause no symptoms in their early stages. This is why screening is essential. Diagnosis relies mainly on two tools: PSA (prostate-specific antigen) blood tests and digital rectal examinations, often followed by a biopsy in cases of suspicion. Symptoms generally appear at a more advanced stage, and include difficulty in urinating, a reduced urine stream, a sensation of incomplete bladder emptying, and sometimes pain in the lower back or pelvis.

Treatment of prostate cancer varies according to the stage of the disease and the patient's age. In the early stages, active surveillance may be proposed if the tumor is small and not very aggressive. For more advanced forms, options include surgery (prostatectomy), radiotherapy or hormone therapy. Support for prostate cancer patients goes far beyond physical care: the psychological impact, particularly in view of possible side effects such as incontinence or erectile dysfunction after treatment, is often profound. The caregiver plays an essential role in helping these men to overcome the difficulties associated with treatment, while ensuring that their dignity is preserved and offering them emotional support during this ordeal.

Bladder cancer is another frequent urological pathology, affecting both men and women, although men are more often affected. It develops from cells in the inner lining of the bladder and is generally linked to risk factors such as smoking or exposure to certain chemicals. The most common symptoms include blood in the urine (hematuria), often painless at first, pain on urination and a frequent urge to urinate. As these symptoms are sometimes associated with urinary tract infections, they can be overlooked or misinterpreted, delaying diagnosis.

Treatment of bladder cancer depends on the stage of the disease. For superficial tumors, endoscopic resection (cystoscopy) may suffice. In more advanced cases, chemotherapy, radiotherapy or even cystectomy (removal of the bladder) may be required. The latter is a particularly invasive treatment, often involving the creation of a urinary shunt, which has a major impact on the patient's quality of life. Caregivers have a crucial role to play in post-operative care, helping patients to adapt to a new way of managing their urinary evacuation. He or she must also support them through the moments of uncertainty and anxiety that often accompany such radical treatment.

Finally, **renal failure** is a pathology that affects the kidneys' ability to filter blood properly and eliminate waste from the body. It can be acute (occurring suddenly and often reversible) or chronic (progressing slowly and irreversibly). There are many causes of renal failure: diabetes, hypertension, repeated kidney infections, or prolonged use of certain nephrotoxic drugs. Symptoms of chronic renal failure include fatigue, edema (water retention), difficulty urinating, nausea and poorly controlled hypertension. In its advanced stages, this disease can lead to a toxic accumulation of waste products in the blood, necessitating heavy treatment such as dialysis or kidney transplantation.

Caregivers play a fundamental role in the day-to-day management of patients with renal failure. They ensure compliance with strict diets, monitor hydration and signs of fluid overload (such as edema or difficulty breathing), and prepare patients for dialysis sessions. As part of the dialysis process, the caregiver helps to set up and monitor patients, ensuring their comfort during this long and often trying procedure. They also provide vital moral support, as chronic renal failure often imposes radical changes on the patient's lifestyle, sometimes resulting in significant emotional distress.

∘   Urinary tract infections: cystitis, pyelonephritis

Urinary tract infections (UTIs), particularly **cystitis** and **pyelonephritis**, are common pathologies in urology that mainly affect the urinary system, and can cause uncomfortable and sometimes serious symptoms if not treated in time. They most frequently affect women, but can also occur in men, especially in later life. Understanding the difference between these infections and how to manage them is essential to ensure effective treatment and prevent complications.

Cystitis is the most common urinary tract infection, especially in women, due to the short length of their urethra, which facilitates the migration of bacteria to the bladder. It is caused by bacteria, mainly **Escherichia coli**, which originate in the digestive tract and colonize the urethra before migrating up to the bladder. Classic symptoms of cystitis include burning or pain on urination, frequent urination even when the bladder is empty, and cloudy or odorous urine. Occasionally, traces of blood may appear in the urine (hematuria). Although often benign, cystitis can be very uncomfortable and can disrupt a patient's quality of life.

The treatment of cystitis is mainly based on antibiotics for a few days, accompanied by recommendations to drink plenty of water to help eliminate the bacteria. In some patients, cystitis may become recurrent, necessitating closer medical follow-up to identify risk factors or anatomical anomalies that could favor repeated infections. Care of cystitis involves ensuring the patient's comfort, monitoring the frequency and quality of urination, and ensuring that hydration instructions are followed.

In some cases, if cystitis isn't properly treated or if it's neglected, the infection can travel back to the kidneys and cause **pyelonephritis**, a much more serious infection affecting kidney tissue. The symptoms of pyelonephritis are more intense than those of simple cystitis. They include high fever, chills, back pain on the side of the affected kidney, as well as nausea and vomiting. Urine may also be cloudy, with signs of hematuria, but the main symptom that differentiates it from simple cystitis is the intense pain in the lower back, at the level of the kidneys.

Pyelonephritis requires prompt treatment, as a kidney infection can lead to serious complications, such as sepsis or permanent kidney damage. Treatment usually involves antibiotics, often intravenous in severe cases, and may require hospitalization, especially if the patient shows signs of dehydration or systemic infection. As a caregiver, monitoring the patient's vital signs (temperature, blood pressure, heart rate) and symptoms is paramount, in order to detect any worsening of the condition and ensure a rapid medical response.

Caregivers also play a key role in prevention, notably by educating patients on the importance of hydration, intimate hygiene, and the behaviors to adopt to avoid recurrences. For women, tips such as urinating after intercourse, adopting gentle hygiene and avoiding irritating products are often recommended to reduce the risk of cystitis. In older people, especially men, the presence of urinary disorders linked to benign prostatic hypertrophy can lead to urine stagnating in the bladder, increasing the risk of infection. In such cases, the caregiver can help monitor urine flow and educate the patient about preventive measures.

  ◦   Urinary incontinence: causes and consequences

Urinary incontinence is a common but often misunderstood and underestimated condition affecting millions of people worldwide. It is characterized by the involuntary loss of urine, a symptom that can have a significant impact on the quality of life of sufferers. Urinary incontinence can affect people of any age, although it is more common in the elderly and in women, particularly after menopause or childbirth. Its causes are multiple and vary according to the type of incontinence, but its consequences, both physical and psychological, are often severe, impacting not only the patient's health, but also his or her emotional and social well-being.

There are several types of urinary incontinence, the **causes of** which vary according to the mechanisms involved. **Stress incontinence** is one of the most common, particularly in women. It occurs when the pressure exerted on the bladder (when coughing, sneezing, exerting physical effort, or simply standing up) exceeds the resistance of the urethral sphincter, causing urine to leak. This type of incontinence is often caused by a weakening of the pelvic floor muscles, which can occur after pregnancies, multiple births, or as a result of aging. In men, prostatectomy (removal of the prostate gland) can sometimes result in stress incontinence, due to damage to the urethral sphincter during surgery.

Urge incontinence is another common type. It manifests itself as a sudden, intense need to urinate, followed by leakage before the person can even reach the toilet. This incontinence is often linked to an overactive bladder, which contracts inappropriately even when the bladder is not yet full. Causes include neurological disorders such as Parkinson's disease or multiple sclerosis, recurrent urinary tract infections, or bladder irritation due to stones or tumors. Urge incontinence can also be linked to neurological problems affecting communication between the brain and the bladder.

Finally, there are mixed forms of incontinence, where symptoms of stress incontinence and urge incontinence are combined, as well as **overflow incontinence**, which occurs when the bladder does not empty completely and eventually overflows. The latter type is more common in men, mainly due to an obstruction in the prostate (benign prostatic hypertrophy) that prevents complete evacuation of urine.

The **consequences of** urinary incontinence are often far more far-reaching than mere physical discomfort. Although urinary leakage is sometimes perceived as minor, it has a profound impact on patients' daily lives. On a **physical** level, frequent leakage can lead to skin irritation and infection (dermatitis), and increase the risk of urinary tract infections. In the elderly or those with reduced mobility, incontinence can also be a cause of falls, when the patient rushes to the toilet to avoid a leak, risking loss of balance.

Psychologically, the consequences can be even more serious. Urinary incontinence is often a source of shame and embarrassment, leading people to avoid certain social activities, restrict their movements or withdraw from public life for fear of not being able to control their leaks. This social isolation can quickly lead to a loss of self-confidence and even depression. Many people affected by incontinence do not talk about their problem, for fear of being judged, and so delay their medical consultation, aggravating the situation.

The **social impact** of incontinence is therefore considerable. People with incontinence may choose to limit their social interactions, cease physical or sporting activities, or alter their routine to stay close to the toilet, significantly affecting their quality of life. The common stigma attached to incontinence means that many patients are reluctant to seek help, reinforcing their isolation.

Fortunately, **solutions** exist to treat urinary incontinence, and they vary according to the cause and type of incontinence. Treatments range from lifestyle changes (weight loss, reducing caffeine or alcohol intake) to pelvic floor strengthening exercises, such as Kegel **exercises**, which are particularly effective for stress incontinence. Other options include drug treatments, to calm overactive bladder, or medical devices, such as pessaries, which can help support the bladder in women. In some cases, surgery is necessary, particularly for men who have had a prostatectomy or for women suffering from severe incontinence after childbirth.

Urological treatments and procedures
◦   Medical and surgical treatments

Medical and surgical treatments in urology are varied and adapted to the specificities of the pathologies encountered, be they infections, functional disorders, kidney stones or cancers. These treatments aim to relieve symptoms, cure diseases, or improve patients' quality of life when complete cure is not possible. Each approach, whether medical or surgical, is determined by the nature of the disease, its stage of progression, and the patient's individual characteristics.

Medical treatments are often preferred as a first approach in less severe or early-stage urological pathologies. These treatments include **drugs** that directly target the cause or symptoms of the disease. For example, in the case of **urinary tract infections**, antibiotics are the treatment of choice to eliminate the bacteria responsible for the infection. Antibiotics can be administered orally for simple infections, such as cystitis, or intravenously in more serious cases, such as pyelonephritis.

In chronic pathologies such as **benign prostatic hyperplasia (BPH)**, which causes an increase in prostate volume and difficulty in urinating, drug treatments aim to relax the prostate and bladder muscles, or reduce the size of the prostate. Medications used include **alpha-blockers**, which facilitate micturition by relaxing the muscles of the prostate and bladder neck, and **5-alpha-reductase inhibitors**, which reduce the size of the prostate by acting on hormones. These treatments are particularly effective in the early stages of BPH, and can delay or even avoid the need for surgery.

In the case of **overactive bladder disorders** or **urinary incontinence**, anticholinergic drugs or beta-3-agonists may be prescribed to reduce involuntary bladder contractions and decrease the frequent urge to urinate. These medical treatments considerably improve patients' quality of life by limiting episodes of urinary leakage and the urgent need to urinate.

However, when drug treatments are not sufficient, or when the disease is too advanced, **surgical treatment** becomes necessary. One of the most frequent urological procedures is **prostatectomy**, which involves the total or partial removal of the prostate gland. It is performed in cases of **benign prostate hyperplasia** resistant to medical treatment, or in cases of **prostate cancer**. Radical prostatectomy, used to treat localized prostate cancer, can be performed by open or laparoscopic surgery, or with the assistance of robotic surgery. The latter technique is more precise and less invasive, enabling faster recovery and limiting the risk of complications such as incontinence or erectile dysfunction.

In the case of **bladder cancer**, surgical treatment depends on the stage of the tumour. If the tumour is superficial, it can be removed by **transurethral resection of the bladder** (TURB), a minimally invasive procedure that removes the tumour through the urethra without incision. For more advanced cancers, a **cystectomy** (total removal of the bladder) may be necessary, accompanied by a urinary diversion to enable the patient to eliminate urine. This major surgery has a major impact on quality of life, and post-operative support is essential to help the patient adapt to this new reality.

Another type of surgery frequently used in urology is the treatment of **urinary lithiasis**, or kidney stones. When the stones are too large to be evacuated naturally, techniques such as **extracorporeal shock wave lithotripsy** (ESWL) are used to break them up so that they can be expelled more easily through the urinary tract. If this technique is not sufficient, **ureteroscopy** or **percutaneous nephrolithotomy** (a direct cutaneous procedure) can be performed to remove the stones. These procedures provide rapid relief from the intense pain and complications associated with kidney stones, such as recurrent urinary tract infections or urinary tract obstruction.

In the event of **end-stage renal failure**, where the kidneys can no longer filter blood efficiently, **dialysis** becomes indispensable. There are two types of dialysis: **hemodialysis**, where blood is filtered outside the body through a machine, and **peritoneal dialysis**, where dialysis fluid is introduced into the abdominal cavity to absorb waste before being drained. Dialysis is a restrictive and burdensome treatment for patients, but it enables life to be maintained while awaiting an eventual **kidney transplant**, which is the treatment of choice for patients with severe chronic renal failure.

       ∘   Different types of catheter (ureteral, suprapubic, etc.)

Urinary catheters play a crucial role in the management of urological disorders and surgical procedures. They enable urine to be drained when the patient is unable to urinate normally, whether due to pathology, urinary tract obstruction or surgery. There are several types of catheter, each adapted to specific clinical situations, and the choice of catheter type depends on the patient's individual needs as well as the expected duration of use. Among the most common are **ureteral**, **suprapubic** and **intermittent** catheters, each with its own indications and modes of insertion.

The **ureteral catheter** is inserted directly into the urethra to reach the bladder and enable the evacuation of urine. This is the type of catheter most frequently used in hospitals, notably in post-operative care, or for patients suffering from urinary retention. It is generally made of latex or silicone and connected to a drainage bag. This type of catheter is often placed after urological surgery, such as prostatectomy or kidney stone surgery, or when a patient is immobilized and unable to use the toilet. Ureteral catheter insertion is generally quick and minimally invasive, but as it is in direct contact with the urethra, it can cause irritation or infection if hygiene is not scrupulously observed. To prevent urinary tract infections associated with its use, it's crucial to maintain good asepsis when inserting it, and to regularly monitor the area for any signs of inflammation or infection.

The **suprapubic catheter**, on the other hand, is inserted directly through the skin, just above the pubic bone, to reach the bladder without passing through the urethra. This procedure is generally performed under local anaesthetic and is used when insertion of a urethral catheter is impossible or inappropriate, for example in cases of urethral obstruction or after trauma to the urethra. The suprapubic catheter is often preferred for patients requiring long-term urinary drainage, as it is more comfortable than the ureteral catheter and reduces the risk of urinary tract infections, since it does not cross the urethra. This type of catheter is also used in patients suffering from neurological pathologies affecting bladder function, such as multiple sclerosis or spinal cord injury, to ensure efficient urine drainage. It improves patient mobility and is easier to manage at home.

Intermittent catheters, also known as **self-lubricating catheters**, are used for **intermittent catheterization**, a technique which involves inserting the catheter several times a day to empty the bladder, then removing it after each use. This type of catheter is often recommended for patients able to catheterize themselves, or with the help of a caregiver. It is particularly suitable for people with chronic urinary retention who have residual bladder function and can avoid the need for a permanent catheter. Intermittent catheterization has the advantage of considerably reducing the risk of infection, since the bladder is left free between catheterizations, unlike permanent catheters which remain in place and provide an entry point for bacteria. Intermittent catheters are often recommended for patients suffering from bladder neuropathy, spinal cord injury or after certain pelvic surgeries.

In addition to these main types of catheter, there are **balloon catheters**, which have a small balloon inflated at the tip, once in the bladder, to prevent the catheter from slipping out. This device is commonly used with ureteral and suprapubic catheters to ensure they stay in place, particularly when the patient needs to be catheterized over a long period.

Each type of catheter has its advantages and disadvantages, and the choice of device depends not only on the patient's medical condition, but also on his or her lifestyle and ability to manage a catheter. Prolonged use of catheters, particularly ureteral and suprapubic catheters, requires constant attention to prevent complications such as urinary tract infections, skin lesions or the formation of bladder stones. The caregiver's role in catheter management is crucial: he or she must ensure rigorous hygiene, regular emptying of drainage bags, monitoring for signs of infection (such as fever, pain or foul-smelling urine), and educating the patient to understand how to care for his or her catheter, especially if it is used at home.

Finally, it's important to note that the use of catheters, although often essential, can have an emotional impact on patients, especially those who have to live with a catheter for the long term. The caregiver therefore also plays an important role in the psychological support of the patient, helping him/her to adapt to

46

this new reality and ensuring that he/she retains maximum autonomy and dignity in his/her daily management.

- ◦ Lithotripsy, prostatectomy, nephrectomy, cystoscopy

In urology, several surgical or medical interventions are essential to treat specific pathologies. Among these, **lithotripsy**, **prostatectomy**, **nephrectomy** and **cystoscopy** are frequently used procedures, each responding to different needs, from the treatment of kidney stones to the management of prostate or kidney cancer. Each of these procedures has its own indications, techniques and implications for patients, and the role of the caregiver is crucial in the preparation and post-operative follow-up of these procedures.

Lithotripsy is a non-invasive technique used to treat **kidney stones** or **urinary calculi**, also known as lithiasis. Stones form in the kidneys or urinary tract from mineral deposits that clump together, and can cause intense pain when they block the flow of urine. Lithotripsy involves using **shock waves** to break up these stones into small pieces, so that they can be evacuated naturally through the urinary tract. There are two main types of lithotripsy: **extracorporeal shock wave lithotripsy** (ESWL), in which waves are emitted from outside the body and directed at the stones, and **endoscopic lithotripsy**, in which an endoscope is inserted to enable direct intervention. The advantage of lithotripsy is that it avoids invasive surgery, reducing recovery time and the risk of complications. The role of the caregiver in this procedure is to prepare the patient prior to the procedure, follow up to ensure stone fragments are removed, and monitor for possible complications, such as infection or urinary retention.

Prostatectomy is a surgical procedure designed to remove all or part of the **prostate**, usually in response to **prostate cancer** or **benign prostatic hyperplasia** (BPH). There are several types of prostatectomy, the most common being **radical prostatectomy**, in which the prostate is completely removed, often accompanied

47

by the seminal vesicles and sometimes the surrounding lymph nodes, to prevent the spread of cancer. This procedure can be carried out in the conventional, open way, or using less invasive techniques such as **laparoscopic** or **robot-assisted surgery**, which reduce incisions, recovery time, and the risk of post-operative complications such as urinary incontinence or erectile dysfunction. **Simple prostatectomy**, on the other hand, is used to treat BPH, and involves removing only the inner part of the prostate that is causing urinary obstruction. The caregiver plays an essential role in preparing the patient prior to the operation, helping him or her to understand the procedure and its implications, as well as ensuring rigorous post-operative follow-up, monitoring recovery and accompanying the patient in managing side effects, such as managing a temporary catheter or perineal rehabilitation to reduce incontinence problems.

Nephrectomy is a major surgical procedure to remove all or part of a **kidney**. It is usually performed in cases of **kidney cancer**, large benign tumors, or when a kidney has been severely damaged by disease or trauma. Nephrectomy can be **total** (the whole kidney is removed) or **partial** (only part of the kidney is removed, usually to preserve remaining kidney function). As with prostatectomy, nephrectomy can be performed openly or by **laparoscopy**, a less invasive technique that allows for faster recovery. Removing a kidney or part of it is a delicate operation, as the kidneys play an essential role in blood filtration and waste elimination. After the operation, the remaining kidney must compensate for the loss of function. The caregiver is particularly involved in post-operative follow-up, monitoring signs of infection, bleeding and kidney function. He or she also helps the patient adapt to his or her new condition, explaining the importance of a rigorous lifestyle to preserve the remaining kidney, in particular by monitoring diet and hydration.

Cystoscopy, on the other hand, is a **diagnostic** and sometimes **therapeutic** procedure that explores the inside of the **bladder** and **urethra** using a **cystoscope**, a thin, flexible tube fitted with a camera. This procedure is used to examine bladder abnormalities,

48

diagnose diseases such as **bladder cancer**, or treat certain problems, such as the resection of small tumors or the removal of bladder stones. Cystoscopy can be performed under **local** or **general anaesthetic**, depending on the extent of the procedure. It is often well tolerated, and enables direct visualization of the bladder wall and lower urinary tract. The caregiver accompanies the patient before the procedure, reassuring him or her and preparing the necessary equipment. After the procedure, he or she monitors the patient's return to normal urinary function, making sure there is no abnormal pain or bleeding, and encouraging the patient to drink plenty of water to flush the bladder.

Chapter 3

Daily management of urology patients

The key role of hygiene and asepsis

∘ Preventing nosocomial infections

The **prevention of nosocomial infections**, i.e. infections contracted during a stay in hospital or any other healthcare establishment, is a crucial issue in the medical environment, and particularly in urology. These infections, which mainly affect vulnerable patients or those undergoing medical or surgical procedures, can have serious consequences, prolonging hospital stays, increasing healthcare costs and, above all, compromising patient health and safety. The nursing auxiliary plays a central role in this prevention, by applying strict hygiene and sterilization protocols, carefully monitoring for signs of infection, and educating patients on preventive measures.

Nosocomial infections are most often caused by **bacteria, viruses** or fungi that develop in the hospital environment, notably as a result of invasive care, medical devices (such as urinary catheters), or contact with contaminated surfaces or equipment. In urology, where patients are often catheterized or undergo surgery, infection prevention is particularly important. Catheter-associated urinary tract infections (also known as **urinary device-associated urinary tract infections**) are among the most frequent nosocomial infections. They can occur when bacteria enter the urinary tract via the catheter, or as a result of inadequate hygiene during catheter insertion and maintenance.

Hand disinfection is one of the first steps in preventing nosocomial infections. All healthcare professionals, including orderlies, must wash their hands rigorously and frequently, before and after each contact with a patient, after touching medical equipment, or after handling a device such as a catheter. The use of hydroalcoholic solutions or antiseptic soap is a basic but essential measure to limit the spread of pathogens. Although essential, this simple and effective measure must be strictly observed to avoid cross-transmission between patients, particularly in high-risk departments such as urology, where the use of invasive devices is commonplace.

Adherence to aseptic techniques during medical procedures is also fundamental to preventing nosocomial infections. This includes using sterile equipment, disinfecting the skin before inserting any catheter or probe, and using sterile gloves and gowns for the caregivers involved in these procedures. When inserting a urinary catheter, for example, it is crucial to follow a strict sterility protocol, using a sterile field, gloves and appropriate disinfection of the surrounding areas. The nursing auxiliary, who often prepares and assists with these procedures, must ensure that these rules are applied correctly, to minimize the risk of introducing bacteria into the urinary tract.

The maintenance of existing **medical devices**, such as urinary catheters, is another potential source of nosocomial infections, and their careful management is paramount. For patients with long-term catheters, it is essential to ensure that the drainage bag is placed below the level of the bladder, to avoid any urine reflux that could introduce bacteria into the urinary tract. Regular emptying of the bag must be carried out under strict hygienic conditions, and drainage circuits must be handled with care to avoid any risk of contamination. The caregiver, who regularly monitors these devices, must be alert to signs of infection (fever, pain, cloudy or foul-smelling urine) and intervene rapidly if infection is suspected.

In addition to medical devices, **disinfection of surfaces** and surrounding equipment is another essential measure for limiting nosocomial infections. In the hospital environment, surfaces such as door handles, beds, or shared equipment (like blood pressure monitors or thermometers) can be vectors for pathogen transmission. Regular cleaning, using appropriate disinfectants, is necessary to reduce the microbial load on these surfaces. Caregivers, who are in direct contact with patients and equipment, must ensure the cleanliness of the care environment, the proper management of medical waste, and the appropriate use of personal protective equipment (gloves, masks) when necessary.

Finally, an often overlooked aspect of nosocomial infection prevention is the **education of patients and their families**. Caregivers play a key role in informing and educating patients about essential hygiene practices, such as hand-washing and managing medical devices in the home. It's important that patients understand how to prevent infection, especially when they return home with a catheter or urinary catheter. Informing relatives and caregivers about good practice is just as crucial, as they are often involved in the patient's day-to-day care. Good education helps reduce the risk of infection once the patient has left hospital.

○   Sterile care techniques (probes, catheters)

Sterile care techniques, particularly for the insertion and management of catheters, are essential to prevent infections and ensure patient safety in the hospital environment. In urology, where invasive devices such as **urinary catheters** are frequently used, rigorous mastery of sterility protocols is essential. When correctly applied, these techniques minimize the risk of contamination by pathogens, thereby reducing the risk of nosocomial infections which can complicate patient recovery.

One of the most important aspects of sterile care is the **careful preparation** of equipment and personnel prior to the procedure. Before handling any catheter or probe, it is crucial that all equipment is sterile. This includes gloves, surgical drapes, instruments and the medical devices themselves. All sterile care begins with hand washing, an essential step in reducing the microbial load on the skin. Caregivers must then put on sterile gloves and ensure that the operating field is clean and delimited by sterile drapes to avoid contamination. This preparation process ensures that every procedure performed complies with sterility standards, thus limiting the risk of introducing bacteria or other infectious agents.

The **insertion of a urinary catheter** is a typical example where sterile care techniques are essential. During this procedure, a catheter is inserted into the urethra to reach the bladder and enable urine to be evacuated. Before inserting the catheter, the urethra and surrounding areas must be carefully disinfected, using a suitable antiseptic solution. It is essential to proceed methodically, avoiding any contact between sterile equipment and non-sterile surfaces. The catheter itself must remain sterile until it is inserted, and particular care must be taken when handling the probe to ensure it does not accidentally touch contaminated surfaces before being introduced into the body. Once the probe is in place, the caregiver must check that the balloon is properly inflated and that the probe is correctly secured, while maintaining impeccable hygiene.

The **management of venous catheters**, although more the concern of other medical specialties, follows similar principles. Whether for **peripheral** or **central catheters**, the procedure begins with the preparation of a sterile operating field around the insertion site, and the application of an antiseptic to the patient's skin. The catheter is inserted using sterile gloves and precise techniques to minimize the risk of infection. After catheter insertion, the insertion site must be protected by a sterile dressing, which must be changed regularly following strict aseptic procedures. Monitoring the insertion site is crucial to detect any signs of infection, such as redness, swelling or discharge.

Once in place, **catheter** management also requires rigorous care to maintain sterility and prevent infection. For example, for **urinary catheters**, it is essential that the drainage bag remains below the level of the bladder to avoid urine reflux, which could introduce bacteria into the urinary tract. The drainage circuit must be handled with care, and the valves emptied aseptically to limit any risk of contamination. In addition, the replacement of catheters at regular intervals, or when medically necessary, must always be carried out using the same sterile techniques as for the initial installation.

The importance of **sterile care techniques** is also evident in the prevention of **catheter-related infections**, which are among the most frequent nosocomial infections. For venous catheters, sterility must be maintained throughout use, whether for infusion or blood sampling. Caregivers must always disinfect connectors and valves before each manipulation, and use single-use or sterilized equipment. Similarly, for urinary catheters, drainage bag changes, emptying and care around the catheter must be carried out according to strict protocols to avoid bacterial colonization.

Another essential aspect of catheter and catheter management is **continuous monitoring** for signs of infection. This includes regular checks of the skin around the insertion site (for catheters) or urethra (for catheters), looking for redness, swelling, pain or unusual secretions. If infection is suspected, it's crucial to intervene quickly, removing the device if necessary and administering an appropriate course of antibiotics. Communication between the various members of the medical team is also essential to ensure effective management and avoid complications.

◦   Hand washing and equipment preparation

Hand-washing and **equipment preparation** are two essential pillars of infection prevention, particularly in hospitals. These simple yet rigorously supervised gestures minimize the risk of micro-organism transmission between caregivers and patients, while ensuring a sterile environment for medical and surgical care. Their importance is particularly crucial in departments such as urology, where procedures often involve sensitive areas, and where invasive devices such as catheters are frequently used.

Hand washing is undoubtedly the first line of defense against nosocomial infections. It is a basic gesture which, although simple, must be carried out rigorously and at key times to be effective. There are two types of handwashing: **simple handwashing** with soap and water, and **antiseptic handwashing**, using hydroalcoholic solutions or disinfectants. Each has its own specific indications, but both aim to eliminate micro-organisms present on the hands before any contact with the patient, sterile equipment or a critical care area.

Hand washing is essential at several stages of care: **before and after any direct contact with a patient**, before handling invasive medical devices (such as urinary catheters), after touching potentially contaminated surfaces or objects, and after removing gloves. Although gloves provide a protective barrier, they are not a substitute for hand washing, as microcracks in gloves or improper handling can introduce germs. Furthermore, washing hands before putting on gloves is crucial to ensure that no bacteria are trapped underneath, increasing the risk of infection.

Simple hand **washing** should be done with liquid soap and lukewarm water, rubbing hands for at least 30 seconds. It's essential not to neglect certain areas, such as the spaces between the fingers, the backs of the hands, the thumbs, and under the fingernails. Hand drying, often neglected, is also an important step: hands should be dried with single-use paper towels or hot air systems, as damp hands are more conducive to the spread of germs. If washing with soap and water is not possible, the use of **hydroalcoholic solutions** is an effective alternative. They are particularly practical in hospital environments, as they enable rapid disinfection and do not require access to a water point.

In addition to hand washing, the **preparation of equipment** used during care plays an equally decisive role in ensuring patient safety. Whether for surgery, invasive care such as urinary catheterization, or lighter procedures, equipment preparation must follow strict sterilization protocols. Medical equipment, whether forceps, probes, catheters or surgical drapes, must be carefully sterilized before use to ensure that they do not carry micro-organisms that could infect the patient.

Equipment sterilization is a process that eliminates not only bacteria, but also viruses and fungal spores. It can be carried out using several techniques, including autoclaving (using pressurized steam), dry heat, or chemical processes, depending on the nature of the equipment. Caregivers must ensure that all materials they use come from **sterile blisters** (sterile packaging), which must only be opened when they are to be used, to maintain their sterility. If reusable equipment is used, it must be processed by the sterilization department before being reused, and its traceability must be rigorously ensured to guarantee that it has followed the appropriate sterilization circuit.

In addition, **preparing the sterile field** is a crucial step in sterile care, particularly during surgery or the insertion of invasive devices. Before installing a catheter or probe, it is essential to establish a sterile zone around the insertion site, using sterile drapes or surgical drapes. This physical barrier limits cross-contamination between non-sterile areas of skin and sterile instruments. Caregivers in charge of equipment preparation must ensure that this sterility barrier is never broken, by scrupulously respecting instrument handling procedures, using sterile gloves and avoiding any contact between sterile equipment and non-sterile surfaces.

Finally, as part of **infection prevention**, caregivers must also make patients and their families aware of the importance of hand-washing, particularly in units where invasive devices are present. Explanatory posters or **demonstrations** on handwashing and the importance of not touching medical devices without precautions can go a long way towards reducing the risk of infection. This education is all the more important when patients go home with catheters, as managing these devices outside the hospital requires extra vigilance on hygiene rules.

Basic and technical care
   ◦ Intimate hygiene and specific hygiene care
Intimate hygiene and **specific hygienic care** are essential elements of patient care in the hospital environment, particularly in departments such as urology, where pathologies and interventions directly affect the genitourinary organs. This care is not only important to ensure patient **comfort** and **dignity**, but also to prevent complications, such as **infections** that can arise from

manipulations or invasive devices like urinary catheters. Intimate hygiene requires a delicate and respectful approach, while complying with strict hygiene and safety standards.

Properly performed, **intimate hygiene** helps to keep perineal areas clean and prevent the build-up of bacteria that can lead to urinary tract or skin infections. It is particularly important for bedridden patients, the elderly, or those suffering from incontinence or wearing urinary catheters. These people are more vulnerable to infection, and their inability to look after their own personal hygiene calls for extra vigilance on the part of the caregiver.

The first step in intimate hygiene is to **respect** the patient's **modesty** and **dignity**. Before starting, it's important to explain the procedure to the patient, even if he or she is unconscious or unable to respond. This establishes a climate of trust and ensures that the patient is at ease. It is also advisable to use a **screen** or close the door to guarantee the patient's privacy, and to uncover only those parts of the body necessary for grooming to minimize exposure.

Equipment preparation is crucial to ensuring hygienic and effective care. The caregiver must have **non-sterile gloves** on hand, as well as gentle cleaning products such as cleansing lotions or impregnated wipes adapted to sensitive areas, and sterile compresses if the grooming involves caring for a particularly sensitive area, such as around a urinary catheter. For patients suffering from allergies or with fragile skin, it's important to choose suitable products, free from perfumes or irritants. The use of lukewarm water is also recommended, as it is more pleasant for the patient and avoids skin irritation.

When cleansing the intimate area, it's essential to follow **precise gestures** to avoid contamination. The basic principle is always to clean from front to back, especially for women, to avoid bringing bacteria from the anal region to the urethra or genitals, which could lead to infection. In men, grooming should include thorough cleaning of the foreskin (if present) and glans, especially if the patient is probed or has undergone urological surgery. The foreskin must be folded back carefully, and once cleansing is complete, the foreskin must be repositioned correctly to avoid the risk of para-phimosis (strangulation of the glans by the foreskin).

For patients with **urinary catheters**, intimate hygiene requires special attention to prevent **infections associated with these devices**. The area around the catheter insertion should be carefully cleaned daily with a mild, sterile solution, and the catheter itself should be handled with clean gloves to prevent the introduction of bacteria. It is also crucial to check the condition of the skin around the catheter for any irritation or signs of infection, such as redness, swelling or secretions. Urine catheter bag management must also follow strict hygiene protocols, with regular emptying and monitoring of urine color and odor, which can provide clues to a developing infection.

Specific hygiene care is also important for patients suffering from **incontinence**. Urinary or faecal incontinence can lead to skin irritation and even bedsores if not properly managed. For these patients, regular cleansing and the use of barrier creams to protect the skin from urine or faeces are essential. Frequent changes of absorbent pads and sheets also help prevent irritation and maintain good body hygiene.

In certain situations, such as after **urological surgery** or **childbirth**, intimate hygiene takes on even greater importance. Sutures, incisions or healing areas must be cleaned with sterile products and following rigorous asepsis techniques to avoid infection. Caregivers must take care not to rub these delicate areas, but rather to gently dab them with sterile compresses soaked in a mild antiseptic solution. Wound monitoring is essential to detect any abnormalities, such as discharge, excessive heat or abnormal redness, which could indicate infection.

Finally, the **psychological** aspect of intimate hygiene should not be overlooked. For many patients, depending on a caregiver for this care can be a source of embarrassment or emotional discomfort. The caregiver must demonstrate kindness, discretion and empathy, ensuring that every gesture is carried out with respect and consideration for the patient's sensitivity. Active listening and attention to the patient's reactions enable care to be adapted to make it more comfortable and less psychologically invasive.

○   Monitoring drains and probes

Monitoring drains and catheters is an essential task in nursing, particularly in urology, where these devices are commonly used after surgical procedures or for the management of certain chronic pathologies. Drains and probes play a crucial role in the evacuation of body fluids, whether urine, secretions or post-operative fluids, and their proper functioning is essential to avoid serious complications, such as infections or obstructions. Careful, regular monitoring of these devices enables potential problems to be detected early, ensuring patient safety and comfort.

Urinary catheters, like bladder catheters, are widely used in urology, either to drain urine when the patient is unable to urinate, or as part of post-operative recovery after procedures such as prostatectomy or bladder surgery. Monitoring a urinary catheter begins with an inspection of the catheter's **secure attachment** and **insertion area**. The caregiver must check that the catheter is properly secured to prevent accidental displacement, and ensure that it does not exert excessive pressure on the urethra, which could cause injury or discomfort. The area around the insertion should be clean and free from redness, swelling or secretions, early signs of infection. Regular cleaning of the area around the catheter with a mild antiseptic solution is recommended to prevent infection, taking care to maintain impeccable hygiene.

Another key aspect of catheter monitoring is **urine flow control**. The caregiver must ensure that urine flows freely through the catheter, and that the **collection bag** is positioned below bladder level to avoid reflux. Low or absent flow may indicate catheter blockage, torsion or obstruction by debris or clots. In this case, it's essential to intervene quickly by adjusting the catheter position or contacting the healthcare team for a replacement if necessary. The color, clarity and odor of urine must also be closely monitored, as changes may indicate an infection or other complication, such as hematuria (blood in the urine) or urinary tract infection. Careful monitoring of these factors helps to prevent and identify possible complications in good time, while ensuring continuous, effective drainage.

Surgical drains, meanwhile, are often used after urological operations to evacuate excess fluids, such as blood, pus or other secretions, accumulated around the operated area. These drains, whether passive or active (such as Redon drains, connected to suction), require regular monitoring to ensure they are working properly and avoid postoperative infections. The caregiver must check several times a day that the drain is in good condition, properly positioned and unobstructed. The drain insertion site should be inspected for signs of infection, such as redness, swelling or purulent discharge. Any change in the appearance of the wound or a sudden increase in the volume of secretions should be reported immediately, as they may indicate a complication, such as infection or haemorrhage.

The **volume and nature of drained fluids** are also important indicators of the progress of postoperative recovery. The caregiver should regularly record the amount of fluid drained, as well as its appearance (clear, cloudy, bloody, purulent), as any abnormal variation may indicate an underlying problem requiring medical intervention. For example, a sudden increase in fluid volume could be a sign of internal bleeding, while purulent fluid may indicate an infection. Similarly, lack of drainage, or an abrupt cessation of flow, may be a sign of a blocked drain or suction device failure, and requires immediate assessment.

The management of **drainage bags** connected to probes or drains is another essential part of monitoring. These bags must be emptied regularly to prevent them from becoming too full, which could lead to reflux and increase the risk of infection. Emptying must be carried out using an aseptic technique, ensuring that the bag outlet never comes into contact with contaminated surfaces, and that the bag is properly resealed after each emptying to maintain sterility. The level of the drainage bag must be constantly monitored to ensure that it remains below the patient's level, in order to promote the smooth flow of fluids.

In addition to the technical aspects, **communication with the patient** is also crucial when monitoring catheters and drains. The caregiver must be alert to **patient complaints**, such as pain, discomfort or burning, which may indicate a problem with the device. It's important to encourage the patient to report any unusual sensations, and to inform them of the importance of monitoring these devices to avoid complications. Sometimes, simply adjusting the patient's position or changing the device's fixation can improve comfort and prevent more serious problems.

Finally, the caregiver plays an essential role **in patient education**, especially for patients returning home with a catheter or drain. It is crucial to explain to patients (and their relatives) how to care for these devices at home, how to empty drainage bags, and what warning signs to look out for to spot an infection or malfunction. The caregiver must ensure that the patient has all the necessary equipment to continue this care at home, and understands the importance of strictly following hygiene and monitoring instructions.

> ○ Post-operative care: scar monitoring, pain management

Postoperative care, particularly in urology, is an essential phase in the recovery process following surgery. Two key aspects of this care are **scar monitoring** and **pain management**, which require constant vigilance on the part of caregivers to ensure optimal healing and prevent complications. This care, although routine, plays a decisive role in the patient's quality of life after surgery and in his or her full recovery.

Scar monitoring after surgery is crucial to prevent and detect infection, promote healing, and ensure that the wound heals in good condition. A surgical wound can be a source of complications if not properly monitored, and signs of infection can quickly develop, particularly around internal scars or visible sutures. The caregiver should examine the scar daily for any abnormalities. A **normal scar** should be clean, without excessive redness, swelling or discharge. If the area around the wound becomes warm to the touch, has significant redness, purulent discharge or increasing pain, this may indicate **infection**. It's vital to act quickly by informing the medical team, so that the appropriate treatment can be given.

Wound **dressings** play a key role in protecting scars. It must be changed regularly, under strict aseptic conditions, to avoid contamination of the wound by outside bacteria. The caregiver must also ensure that the dressing remains dry and clean, as moist or soiled dressings can encourage the proliferation of germs. Modern dressings, which are often adhesive and transparent, make it easier to monitor the scar without having to remove the dressing. However, in the event of dampness under the dressing, as in the case of an accumulation of secretions, it is imperative to change it quickly to avoid maceration, which can delay healing.

Healing also depends on the patient's general condition. Good **nutrition** and adequate **hydration** promote tissue regeneration and accelerate wound closure. The caregiver must ensure that the patient adopts a balanced diet and consumes sufficient fluids, as dehydration or poor nutrition can hinder the healing process. In addition, it is crucial to limit **excessive mobilization of** the operated area. If the scar is located in an area subject to tension (for example, the abdomen or groin after urological surgery), care must be taken to ensure that the patient follows rest instructions and avoids sudden movements that could reopen the wound.

Alongside scar monitoring, **pain management** is an equally fundamental aspect of post-operative care. Pain, if not properly managed, can have a direct impact on the healing process, increasing stress, reducing patient mobility and slowing recovery. The caregiver's job is to monitor pain intensity, using appropriate **assessment** scales (numerical or visual), and to ensure that the prescribed analgesic treatment is correctly administered and effective.

There are several types of treatment for post-operative pain, depending on the nature and severity of the operation. **Level 1 analgesics**, such as paracetamol, are often administered for mild to moderate pain. For more intense pain, particularly after major urological procedures such as prostatectomy or nephrectomy, **Level 2 analgesics** (mild opiates such as codeine) or **Level 3** (morphine and derivatives) may be required. The caregiver must closely monitor the effect of these drugs, ensuring that pain is well controlled and observing for any **side effects**, such as nausea, vomiting or constipation, which are common with opiates.

In addition to medication, other non-pharmacological measures can help **manage pain**. Applying **cold compresses** to the operated area can reduce inflammation and relieve localized pain. The caregiver can also encourage **relaxation** techniques, such as deep breathing, to help the patient better manage pain. It's important to stress that pain is not just physical, but can also have a psychological impact. Active listening and emotional support are essential to help the patient through this difficult phase of recovery.

One of the objectives of pain management is also to enable the patient to gently **mobilize** the operated areas as soon as possible. Early mobilization, even if only slight, is important to prevent complications such as **venous thrombosis** (blood clots) or **bedsores** in bedridden patients. By relieving pain appropriately, the caregiver enables the patient to get up gradually, move around and regain some of his or her independence, while avoiding compromising the healing process.

Communication between patient and caregiver is essential in pain management. Patients must be encouraged to express their sensations, to report any persistent or new pain, and to actively participate in their own relief by following instructions. The caregiver plays a key role in this dynamic, ensuring attentive monitoring, adapting care to the patient's needs and acting as a privileged interlocutor between the patient and the medical team.

Patient comfort and mobility
     ◦   Mobilization assistance after surgery

Assisting mobilization after surgery is a crucial step in patient recovery. Early mobilization, i.e. encouraging the patient to move, stand up and walk as soon as possible after surgery, plays an essential role in preventing complications and promoting rapid recovery. It reduces the risk of **post-operative complications** such as **deep vein thrombosis** (blood clots), **pressure sores** (ulcers) and **respiratory complications** associated with prolonged bed rest. The nursing auxiliary, through its support and supervision, is a key player in this rehabilitation phase, providing both technical assistance and psychological support.

Mobilization must be adapted to the patient's condition, the nature of the surgery, and the progress of his or her convalescence. After urological surgery, such as **prostatectomy**, **nephrectomy** or bladder surgery, pain, fatigue and any medical devices (such as urinary catheters or drains) may restrict the patient's movements. It is therefore important to proceed gradually, taking into account the physical limitations and anxiety the patient may feel about moving around after the operation.

In the hours following surgery, **passive mobilization** can be initiated. This involves helping the patient to change position in bed, by gently lifting his or her legs or helping him or her to turn onto his or her side. This change of position helps prevent **bedsores** and promotes blood circulation. The caregiver can also encourage the patient to perform simple movements, such as **flexing and extending the feet** or **gently moving the legs**, to stimulate circulation and prevent blood clots. These movements, although limited, are essential to avoid **venous stasis** and maintain minimal muscle activity.

Once the patient is stabilized and his/her condition permits, usually within 24 to 48 hours of the operation, **active mobilization** can begin. This involves encouraging the patient to sit upright at the edge of the bed, with the help of the caregiver. This apparently simple act can be a real challenge for the patient, especially if he or she is suffering from post-operative pain or dizziness. The caregiver plays a crucial role here, providing physical support, holding the patient to avoid any imbalance, while verbally encouraging her/him. It is important to proceed slowly and carefully, watching for signs of **discomfort**, such as dizziness, sudden paleness or accelerated heart rate, which may indicate orthostatic hypotension (a drop in blood pressure when moving to a standing position).

Once seated at the edge of the bed, the patient can gradually be encouraged to **get up** and, with the help of the caregiver or a walker, to take a few steps around the room. These first, albeit limited, steps are essential to restore the patient's confidence in his or her ability to move around after the operation. The caregiver must remain attentive to every movement, ensuring that medical devices such as catheters or drains are correctly positioned to avoid traction or discomfort.

As the days go by, the aim is to gradually increase the range of movement and duration of movement. Patients can be encouraged to walk for longer and longer periods, first in their room, then in the corridor, always under supervision. **Regular walking** helps prevent many complications, by improving blood circulation, stimulating intestinal transit (often disrupted after surgery), and promoting lung re-expansion, which helps prevent **respiratory complications** such as pneumonia. What's more, regaining mobility has a positive effect on patient morale, restoring a sense of control and independence.

Pain management is a key factor in facilitating mobilization. Postoperative pain, if not properly relieved, can hinder the patient's willingness to mobilize. The caregiver must therefore ensure that analgesic treatments are properly administered and adapted, so that pain does not become an obstacle to recovery. Non-pharmacological methods, such as applying ice to the operated area or relaxation techniques, can also be used to ease pain and facilitate movement.

The caregiver must also consider the **psychological factors** that can influence mobilization. Some patients may be afraid or anxious about moving around after surgery, for fear of experiencing pain or worsening their condition. In these situations, the role of the caregiver is not limited to the physical aspect, but also involves psychological support. It's important to encourage patients, respond to their concerns, and remind them of the healing benefits of mobilization. A benevolent, reassuring attitude can help overcome this apprehension.

Finally, assistance with mobilization after surgery doesn't stop at the hospital. When the patient returns home, it is often necessary to continue these efforts to regain full mobility. The caregiver, in collaboration with physiotherapists or doctors, must provide the patient and family with **practical advice on** how **to** continue mobilization safely at home. This may include specific exercises, recommendations on frequency of movement, or tips on how to avoid falls. The caregiver also ensures that the patient's home environment is suitable, by removing obstacles and ensuring that the patient has appropriate technical aids (such as a walker or grab bars).

      ◦   Pressure sore prevention and skin monitoring

Pressure sore prevention and **skin monitoring** are top priorities in the care of bedridden or mobility-impaired patients, as pressure sores, also known as **pressure ulcers**, can have serious consequences for the patient's health. Pressure sores form when pressure exerted on certain areas of the body, combined with friction or prolonged immobility, causes a reduction in the blood supply to skin tissue, resulting in skin lesions that can develop into deep wounds. These lesions generally appear on bony areas of the body, such as the heels, hips, sacrum or elbows. Preventing pressure sores requires constant vigilance on the part of the nursing team, regular mobilization of the patient, and careful monitoring of skin condition.

One of the first preventive measures is to **reduce pressure points** in high-risk areas. To achieve this, it is essential to **regularly change the** bedridden patient's **position**. Depending on the patient's condition, it is advisable to change position every two hours to prevent certain areas from withstanding prolonged pressure. The caregiver must mobilize the patient carefully, using appropriate techniques to limit rubbing and shearing, which can aggravate the risk of skin lesions. For example, when it's necessary to lift or turn a patient, the use of **transfer lips** or **sliding sheets** enables the patient to be moved gently, thus reducing friction on the skin.

Special cushions and **mattresses** also play a crucial role in pressure sore prevention. Devices such as **dynamic air mattresses** or **gel pads** distribute pressure evenly over the body, reducing pressure points. These devices are particularly effective for patients at high risk of developing pressure sores, such as those suffering from circulatory disorders or malnutrition. The caregiver must ensure that these devices are used and positioned correctly, regularly adjusting the supports according to the patient's needs.

Regular **skin monitoring** is another essential component of pressure sore prevention. Caregivers should examine bedridden patients' skin daily, especially in high-risk areas, to spot the first signs of pressure sore formation. These signs include persistent redness that does not disappear with pressure (stage 1), areas that are warmer or colder than the rest of the skin, swelling, or areas where the skin becomes softer or harder. Redness that persists after pressure has been relieved is often the first warning sign of a pressure sore. Intervening at this early stage can prevent the lesion from worsening. The caregiver must also be alert to the patient's complaints of tingling or discomfort, which may indicate skin irritation.

Skin hygiene also plays a key role in pressure sore prevention. The skin of bedridden or incontinent patients is particularly vulnerable to irritation, as moisture and the acidity of urine or feces can degrade the skin barrier. It is therefore important to maintain **regular**, gentle **cleansing**, using non-irritating products and **barrier creams** to protect the skin, especially in areas prone to maceration. After each wash, the skin should be thoroughly dried, as moisture encourages the formation of bedsores. For patients suffering from incontinence, it's crucial to change absorbent pads frequently, while ensuring that the skin remains clean and dry.

Nutrition is another key factor in pressure sore prevention. Patients who are malnourished or dehydrated are more likely to develop pressure sores, as their skin is more fragile and heals less well. The caregiver must ensure that the patient receives an adequate and balanced diet, rich in proteins, vitamins and minerals, which are essential for the regeneration of skin tissue. Hydration is just as important: well-moisturized skin is more resistant and less prone to lesions. If necessary, nutritional supplements can be offered to patients with nutritional deficiencies.

If a pressure sore appears, even at an early stage, it's crucial to adapt care immediately. The affected area must be relieved of all pressure, and **specific dressings** can be applied to protect the skin and promote healing. Hydrocolloid dressings, for example, create a moist environment conducive to healing and protect the wound from infectious agents. The caregiver must carefully monitor the wound, taking into account its appearance, depth and any suspicious changes. If the pressure sore worsens, with tissue necrosis or infection, the intervention of a physician or wound care specialist is required to implement more advanced

70

treatments, such as surgical debridement or the application of negative pressure therapies.

Regular mobilization of the patient, even in moderation, is a key factor in pressure sore prevention. Encouraging the patient to move, sit up or change position (when their condition allows) helps to reduce pressure on certain areas and improve blood circulation. The caregiver must collaborate with the medical team and physiotherapists to develop a mobilization plan adapted to the patient's abilities.

     ◦   Patient set-up for examinations and procedures (cystoscopy, radiology)

Setting up the patient for examinations and procedures is an essential step in ensuring patient comfort and safety, while facilitating the performance of the medical act under optimum conditions. Whether it's a **cystoscopy**, **radiology** examination or other urological procedure, the nursing auxiliary plays a fundamental role in the physical and psychological preparation of the patient. Correct positioning not only reduces patient discomfort and anxiety, but also avoids complications associated with poor posture or prolonged immobilization. It is therefore crucial for the caregiver to follow precise protocols, while showing empathy for the patient's individual needs.

During a **cystoscopy**, an invasive urological examination which involves exploring the inside of the bladder and urethra using a cystoscope, patient positioning is a delicate stage. The patient is generally placed in the **gynecological position** on an examination table, with legs slightly apart and supported by stirrups, allowing optimum access to the urethra. The caregiver must ensure that the patient is positioned comfortably and stably, adjusting the stirrups so that the legs are well supported without creating tension in the lower back or hips. Before starting, it's important to **prepare the patient** by explaining the procedure, answering any questions and reassuring him or her about how long it will take and how it may feel during the procedure. Communication is essential to reduce anxiety, especially during an examination perceived as intimate or uncomfortable.

Once the patient is settled in, it is important to ensure that all the necessary equipment is within easy reach of the doctor or medical team, while guaranteeing the **sterility of** the operating field. The caregiver must also ensure that the patient's modesty is protected, by uncovering only those parts of the body necessary for the procedure, and covering the rest of the body with sterile sheets or drapes. Maintaining privacy and dignity is particularly crucial in invasive examinations such as cystoscopy, where the patient may feel vulnerable.

When using a **rigid cystoscope**, it is important to immobilize the patient to prevent any sudden movements during insertion of the instrument. The caregiver must therefore ensure that the patient is well positioned and relaxed. If necessary, the medical team may administer a local anaesthetic or sedative to reduce discomfort, but even in these cases, the caregiver's support remains crucial to adjusting the patient's position and reassuring him/her throughout the examination.

When it comes to **radiology** examinations, whether performed for diagnostic purposes or as part of post-operative follow-up, patient positioning is equally important. Whether for **X-rays**, **CT scans** or **MRIs**, the orderly must ensure that the patient is correctly positioned on the examination table, often in the **supine position**, to guarantee accurate images. In radiology, **standing still** is often required, so it's essential that the patient is installed in a position that is both comfortable and stable, to minimize involuntary movements that could impair the quality of the examination.

For patients suffering from post-operative pain or chronic pathologies such as urological or orthopedic disorders, remaining motionless during an examination can be a difficult ordeal. Caregivers must take care to position **cushions** or **supports** under sensitive areas, such as the lower back or knees, to alleviate pressure points and avoid discomfort. In some cases, straps or special devices can be used to keep the patient in the required position, while ensuring comfort.

Preparing the patient for an X-ray examination also involves **checking that there are no contraindications**, particularly with regard to metallic objects or implanted medical devices. For an MRI examination, for example, it is essential to ensure that the patient is not wearing any metal objects, whether jewelry, removable dental prostheses or medical devices that are incompatible with the MRI's powerful magnetic field. The caregiver should therefore take the time to check these details with the patient before entering the examination room, and explain the importance of this precaution.

In addition to the technical aspects, **psychological** support for the patient is a fundamental aspect of installation for examinations and interventions. Some patients may feel anxious about procedures they are unfamiliar with, or anticipate as painful or uncomfortable. The caregiver must listen to these fears and respond with kindness and clarity to reassure the patient. For example, for an examination such as an MRI, where the patient is enclosed in a tunnel for several minutes, it is essential to explain in advance what he or she will feel, to insist on the absence of pain, and to remind him or her that he or she will be constantly monitored by the medical team. **Relaxation** techniques, such as deep breathing, can also be suggested to help the patient better manage stress.

Finally, after the examination or procedure, the caregiver must help the patient to **settle down properly** to recover. For patients who have undergone local or general anesthesia, or for those who have been in an uncomfortable position for a long time, it is crucial to ensure that they do not feel dizzy or weak before helping them to get up or move around. Physical support and accompaniment during the transition to the bedroom or rest room are essential to avoid any discomfort or falls.

Chapter 4

Emergency management in urology

Recognizing and responding to urological complications

○ Acute urinary retention

Acute urinary retention is a urological emergency characterized by the sudden inability to evacuate urine, despite a full bladder. This condition can cause significant discomfort and severe pain, as urine continues to accumulate in the bladder without being able to be expelled. Acute urinary retention requires prompt treatment to relieve pain and avoid serious complications, such as kidney damage or urinary tract infection. This problem can affect both men and women, although it is much more frequent in men, notably due to prostate-related pathologies.

The causes of acute urinary retention are varied and may include **mechanical** or **functional obstructions** of the urinary tract. One of the most common causes in men is **benign prostatic hyperplasia** (BPH), an enlargement of the prostate gland that compresses the urethra and blocks the passage of urine. This phenomenon is often exacerbated by triggering factors, such as excessive fluid intake, the use of certain medications (anticholinergic or sympathomimetic), or episodes of constipation. In women, acute urinary retention can occur as a result of **pelvic prolapse**, where the pelvic organs descend and compress the urethra, or after certain gynaecological surgeries.

The **symptoms** of acute urinary retention are quickly recognized. The patient complains of an urge to urinate, but is unable to do so. This inability is accompanied by a sensation of painful tension in the lower abdomen, linked to distension of the bladder. To the touch, the abdomen is often hard and bulging above the pubis, a sign of a full, distended bladder. Pain can be intense, increasing the patient's discomfort and requiring immediate intervention to relieve the bladder.

Initial management **of** acute urinary retention involves **draining urine** from the bladder to relieve pain and avoid complications. The most common and rapid method is the insertion of a **urinary catheter** (bladder catheter). The caregiver plays a key role in this procedure, preparing the necessary equipment and supporting the patient throughout. The catheter is generally inserted through the urethra, following strict sterility protocols to prevent infection. Once the catheter is in place, the urine is evacuated, and the patient feels immediate relief. Large volumes of urine, sometimes in excess of a liter, are often evacuated during the first emptying of the bladder.

In some cases, if a urethral catheter is not possible due to obstruction, a suprapubic **catheter can** be inserted. This involves inserting a catheter directly into the bladder through the abdominal wall, under local anaesthetic. This **technique** is used when obstruction is too great for a catheter to pass through the urethra, or when there are contraindications to urethral catheterization.

Once acute urinary retention has been treated by catheterization, the medical team carries out investigations to identify the **underlying cause of** the retention. In addition to the history, a **urological workup** is often performed, including imaging studies such as ultrasound to assess prostate size in men, or to detect pelvic or bladder abnormalities in women. **Urinalysis** is also performed to check for urinary tract infections, which may be the consequence or cause of urinary retention.

Long-term treatment depends on the cause identified. In men suffering from BPH, drug treatments such as **alpha-blockers** are often prescribed to relax the prostate muscles and facilitate urine flow. In more severe cases, surgery may be required to reduce the size of the prostate (transurethral resection of the prostate or prostatectomy). In women, treatment may include measures to correct prolapse or resolve other anatomical causes of obstruction. Sometimes, **perineal rehabilitation** is recommended to strengthen pelvic muscles and help prevent recurrence of retention.

Post-acute **monitoring** is essential. If a urinary catheter has been inserted, the caregiver must ensure that it is working properly, monitoring the color, quantity and odor of the urine, as well as the condition of the insertion site to prevent infection. The patient must be made aware of the warning signs of a recurrence, such as difficulty in urinating, reduced urine flow, or pain in the lower abdomen, and must know when to seek prompt medical attention to avoid further retention.

The **psychological** aspect of acute urinary retention should not be overlooked. The feeling of powerlessness to evacuate urine, and the pain associated with bladder distension, can be very stressful for the patient. The caregiver must show empathy, reassure the patient and explain the steps involved in the treatment, stressing the temporary nature of the situation. Providing sympathetic support reduces anxiety and makes the experience less traumatic for the patient.

 ◦   Severe urinary tract infection: urological sepsis
Severe urinary tract infection, when it progresses to **urological sepsis**, represents a serious medical situation requiring urgent and intensive management. Urological sepsis is a systemic inflammatory response triggered by a urinary tract infection that has spread into the bloodstream, leading to potential organ failure. This condition is often caused by an ascending infection that starts in the lower urinary tract, such as cystitis or pyelonephritis, and becomes complicated when not treated in time or appropriately. Progression to sepsis poses a vital threat, as the bacteria responsible for the infection invade the bloodstream, triggering a generalized inflammatory reaction throughout the body.

The **causes of** urological sepsis are varied, but the main ones include **untreated urinary tract infections**, **urinary tract obstructions** (such as kidney stones or benign prostatic hypertrophy), **prolonged urinary catheterization**, or **surgical procedures** such as catheterization or ureter stenting. These conditions encourage urine stagnation, creating an environment conducive to bacterial proliferation, and facilitating the passage of germs into the bloodstream. The bacteria most often implicated in urological sepsis are **gram-negative bacteria** such as **Escherichia coli**, but other pathogens may also be involved.

The **symptoms** of a severe urinary tract infection progressing to urological sepsis are dramatic and require immediate medical attention. The patient presents classic signs of urinary tract infection, such as pain on urination (dysuria), frequent urination, fever and pain in the lower abdomen or kidneys (lumbago). However, in sepsis, these symptoms are rapidly accompanied by more systemic signs: **high fever** (or sometimes hypothermia), **chills**, **tachycardia** (increased heart rate), **hypotension** (reduced blood pressure), **confusion** or altered consciousness, and in advanced cases, signs of **organ failure**, such as breathing difficulties or reduced urine output.

Urological sepsis develops in several stages. When identified at an early stage, the patient may present with **Systemic Inflammatory Response Syndrome** (SIRS), where inflammation becomes generalized throughout the body. If not promptly managed, the infection progresses to **severe sepsis**, with life-threatening organ failure, including acute renal failure, treatment-refractory hypotension and respiratory failure. In the most severe cases, sepsis progresses to **septic shock**, an absolute emergency in which blood pressure drops dangerously and several organs may cease to function, requiring intensive care.

The **management of urological sepsis** is based on a number of principles, all of which must be implemented as a matter of urgency. Firstly, it is essential to administer **broad-spectrum antibiotics** as soon as sepsis is suspected, without waiting for the results of urine and blood cultures. Treatment is often subsequently adjusted according to the results of the antibiogram to target the specific pathogen. **Antibiotic therapy** should be administered intravenously for rapid action, and in some cases, hospitalization in an intensive care unit is required to closely monitor the patient's vital functions.

In addition to antibiotic therapy, management of urological sepsis also involves **unblocking urinary tract obstructions,** if present. Obstructions may be due to kidney stones, tumors or anatomical anomalies. Draining the bladder and kidneys is crucial to eliminating the infection at source. This may involve placement of a **urinary catheter, ureter stent** or, in more severe cases, **nephrostomy** (direct drainage of the kidney through an opening in the skin). Removing the obstruction reduces pressure in the urinary tract and prevents urine retention, which encourages bacterial proliferation.

Another key aspect of management is **hemodynamic resuscitation** to stabilize the patient. Due to the severe hypotension often associated with septic shock, intravenous fluid infusions are administered to maintain blood pressure and improve circulation. If this is not enough, vasopressor drugs may be required to raise blood pressure and ensure an adequate supply of blood to vital organs.

The role of the caregiver in the management of urological sepsis is crucial, particularly in the continuous monitoring of the patient's condition and in the psychological and physical support he/she provides. They must closely monitor **vital parameters** such as temperature, heart rate, blood pressure and respiratory rate, in collaboration with the nursing team. In addition, the caregiver is often responsible for **monitoring urine**, noting its quantity and appearance, which can provide valuable clues as to the progress of the infection. Any sudden change in the patient's condition, such as a deterioration in consciousness, an increase in fever or a drop in urine output, should be reported immediately to the medical team.

The **psychological** and **emotional** aspects of management must not be overlooked. Urological sepsis is an extremely stressful condition for patients and their families. The caregiver plays an important role in reassuring the patient, explaining the treatment steps and providing a constant, reassuring presence. The fear and anxiety that often accompany such a serious situation can be alleviated by clear explanations and empathetic care.

◦   Post-operative bleeding

Post-operative hemorrhage is a dreaded complication that can occur after surgery and requires rapid, rigorous management. It is characterized by excessive blood loss from the surgical site, which can lead to hemodynamic imbalances, hemorrhagic shock and, in the most serious cases, loss of vital functions. Management of this complication relies on early detection of signs of hemorrhage, continuous patient monitoring and immediate medical intervention.

Post-operative hemorrhage can have many **causes**. It can occur as a result of the failure of sutures or ligature stitches to ensure proper hemostasis (bleeding control) during the operation. In some cases, it may be due to coagulation disorders in the patient, infections, or early movements that place excessive stress on the operated area. Urological procedures, especially those involving vascular-rich organs such as the kidneys, prostate or bladder, are particularly prone to bleeding, due to the complexity of the structures and the proximity of major blood vessels.

The **warning signs** of post-operative bleeding must be carefully monitored by the nursing team. **External bleeding**, visible at the surgical site, is the most obvious sign. This may take the form of continuous oozing or a more abundant flow of bright red blood, indicating active bleeding. Blood-soaked dressings or discharge from sheets must be systematically monitored, and the amount recorded to inform the medical team.

However, not all post-operative hemorrhages are visible. **Internal bleeding** can occur in a body cavity, such as the abdomen or chest, with no apparent external signs. In such cases, the caregiver must be particularly attentive to more subtle symptoms, such as **sudden pallor**, **cold sweat**, a **drop in blood pressure** (hypotension), an **increase in heart rate** (tachycardia) or a

decrease in diuresis (reduced urine output). These signs indicate that blood volume is rapidly decreasing, and that the patient is going into **hemorrhagic shock**.

Depending on the extent of the hemorrhage, the **consequences** can vary. Moderate hemorrhage can result in weakness, dizziness and general malaise, but massive hemorrhage can lead to hemorrhagic shock, a situation where the heart is no longer able to maintain sufficient blood pressure to supply vital organs. Hemorrhagic shock is a life-threatening emergency requiring immediate intervention to restore circulating blood volume and stop the hemorrhage.

Initial management of post-operative bleeding begins with stabilizing the patient. In the event of heavy bleeding, the first step is to apply **local compression** to the surgical site in an attempt to control the bleeding. If internal bleeding is suspected, the patient must be kept under constant surveillance, until the doctor or surgeon arrives to assess the situation.

Fluid resuscitation is an essential step in the management of hemorrhage. The patient receives **intravenous infusions of** solutions to compensate for the loss of blood volume and maintain blood pressure. In more severe cases, a **blood transfusion** may be necessary to replace lost blood and restore hemoglobin levels, essential for transporting oxygen to the organs. The caregiver must ensure that these infusions are administered promptly and that the patient's condition is closely monitored during resuscitation.

When bleeding is due to failure of the surgical site, **further surgery** may be required to stop the bleeding. The surgeon may need to reopen the wound to identify and repair bleeding vessels, or to evacuate an internal hematoma that is compressing surrounding organs. In these situations, the caregiver plays a crucial role in preparing the patient for emergency surgery, by informing the medical team, maintaining vital sign monitoring, and ensuring that the necessary protocols are in place.

Once bleeding has been controlled, **post-hemorrhage monitoring** is just as important to prevent recurrence and manage any complications. The caregiver must keep a close eye on the surgical wound, regularly checking the dressing for any signs of bleeding. **Vital parameters** must be monitored frequently, with careful attention to blood pressure, pulse, temperature and diuresis. It is also important to watch for the appearance of subcutaneous **hematoma** or swelling around the surgical site, which could indicate an undrained accumulation of blood.

Patient recovery from post-operative bleeding can be lengthy, especially if blood transfusion or emergency surgery has been required. Careful monitoring of the patient's general condition is essential, including energy recovery and gradual return to a normal diet. In some cases, additional examinations, such as ultrasound or computed tomography (CT) scans, may be carried out to ensure that there is no residual bleeding.

The **caregiver's role** is not limited to physical monitoring. It also includes a **psychological** aspect, reassuring the patient, who may be very anxious about the possibility of bleeding. The caregiver must clearly explain each stage of care and the procedures to come, while being attentive to signs of emotional distress. This human dimension of care is essential to help the patient get through this unexpected complication with as little stress as possible.

The caregiver's role in the emergency team
   ◦   Managing stress and emotions in emergency situations

Managing stress and emotions in the face of emergencies is a fundamental aspect of working in a medical environment, particularly for caregivers faced with critical situations where patients' lives may be at risk. In an environment where decisions have to be made quickly and pressure is constant, knowing how to manage emotions and stress is essential to ensuring patient safety and maintaining optimum quality of care. Caregivers, such as orderlies, nurses and doctors, are often on the front line when faced with unexpected situations, where self-control and the ability to act calmly and effectively are paramount.

When an **emergency situation** occurs, such as cardiac arrest, massive hemorrhage or anaphylactic shock, stress can manifest itself in a variety of ways. It can lead to physical reactions such as increased heart rate, faster breathing or excessive sweating, as well as psychological reactions such as panic, confusion or paralysis in the face of action. At such moments, stress **management** involves channelling these reactions so as not to let emotions overwhelm our ability to judge and act. The ability to stay focused and act methodically under pressure is a sign of professionalism and emergency preparedness.

One of the first steps in managing stress is to **stay focused on priorities**. When faced with an emergency, it's crucial to focus on the actions that need to be taken immediately, following the emergency protocols that have been learned beforehand. These protocols are designed to guide caregivers in their actions, enabling them to avoid wasting time thinking at a time when every second counts. The **organization of priorities** helps to reduce anxiety linked to the situation, as the caregiver knows exactly what to do at each stage, whether to resuscitate a patient, stabilize a critical condition or call for reinforcements.

Training and **regular rehearsal of emergency procedures** are key tools for effective stress management. By rehearsing these actions in simulated emergencies, caregivers integrate them automatically, enabling them to react more quickly and calmly to real-life situations. The better prepared a caregiver is, the more able they are to manage their emotions in action. Training in resuscitation techniques, the management of hemorrhagic shock and the use of emergency medical equipment all boost self-confidence and reduce feelings of panic in the face of the unexpected.

Another key aspect of emergency stress management is **clear and effective communication** with the medical team. Emergency situations are rarely managed alone; they often involve close collaboration with other members of the healthcare team. Concise, precise and unambiguous communication helps to coordinate efforts and avoid errors. The caregiver, for example, must be able to transmit vital information quickly, such as observed clinical signs (heart rate, blood pressure, state of consciousness), and follow the instructions of the doctor or head nurse. Good communication not only helps streamline actions, but also reduces stress, as everyone knows what they have to do and can concentrate on their specific task.

Controlled breathing is a simple but effective technique for managing stress in emergency situations. By breathing deeply and slowly, caregivers can calm their heart rate and oxygenate their brain, helping them to think more clearly and reduce anxiety. Abdominal breathing, for example, is a widely used method for lowering stress levels in a matter of seconds. Taking a moment to **breathe deeply** before taking action helps you refocus and approach the situation with greater calm and control.

Managing emotions in an emergency context also means knowing how to maintain an **emotional distance while** remaining empathetic. It's natural to feel fear, anxiety or sadness when a patient is in danger, but it's important not to let these emotions take over the action. Professional **compassion** means remaining attentive and human, while maintaining a certain emotional distance that enables you to remain focused on care. It is only after the emergency has passed that the caregiver can give way to a more emotional reflection on what has just happened.

After an emergency situation, it's essential to take the time to **debrief** and **deal with the accumulated stress**. Debriefing allows you to look back on events, discuss what went well and what could have been improved, and **share your emotions** with other team members. Mutual support between colleagues is fundamental to overcoming emergency-related stress. Talking about feelings and experiences helps reduce the emotional burden and prevent burnout or chronic stress.

In a preventive approach, stress management also requires a **balanced lifestyle**. A caregiver who takes care of himself or herself, by maintaining a healthy diet, a good sleep pattern and regular physical activity, will be better able to cope with stressful situations in the medical environment. In addition, long-term **stress management** techniques such as meditation, yoga or relaxation can be highly beneficial in building resilience in difficult situations.

Finally, **adaptability** is a key skill in emergency stress management. Medical emergencies are by definition unpredictable, and it is sometimes necessary to quickly change priorities or improvise in the face of unforeseen circumstances. A caregiver who is able to adapt to circumstances, while remaining calm, will be able to face the most complex situations with serenity.

○   Collaborate effectively with the medical team

Effective collaboration with the medical team is essential to providing quality care and ensuring the safety and well-being of patients. The effectiveness of a medical team depends on fluid communication, a clear division of roles and responsibilities, and a spirit of collaboration that emphasizes complementary skills. Whether in an emergency department, an operating theatre, or a specialized hospital department such as urology, the ability to work in synergy with all healthcare professionals (doctors, nurses, orderlies, physiotherapists, etc.) is essential to guarantee optimum patient care.

One of the first pillars of effective collaboration is **clear, structured communication**. The transmission of accurate, comprehensible information is essential to avoid errors and ensure smooth care. Caregivers need to be able to convey important information about the patient's condition, any changes observed or test results in a concise, straightforward manner. For example, when a caregiver notices signs of deterioration in a patient (pain, breathing difficulties, changes in vital parameters), it is crucial that he or she immediately informs the nurse or doctor with precise details, including the time of onset of symptoms, their intensity and their evolution. **Written communication** in the form of patient records, reports or notes in the medical file must also be rigorous and exhaustive, to enable the team to follow the patient's progress with precision.

In addition to verbal communication, **non-verbal communication** plays an important role in collaboration. Healthcare professionals need to be attentive to the gestures, attitudes and facial expressions of team members, as these can reveal important signals about the seriousness of a situation or the need for urgent intervention. Listening, maintaining a sympathetic gaze and being available are essential aspects of effective non-verbal communication that strengthens team cohesion.

A **clear division of roles and responsibilities** within the medical team is also essential to ensure harmonious collaboration. Each member of the team, whether doctor, nurse, orderly or technician, must have a clear understanding of his or her role and responsibilities in patient care. This helps avoid confusion and redundancy, while ensuring that each task is carried out efficiently. For example, in an emergency situation, the nurse may be responsible for administering medication, while the orderly monitors vital parameters, and the doctor concentrates on diagnosis and decision-making. The right organization of tasks is essential to ensure that the patient receives prompt, appropriate care, without wasting time through poor coordination.

Team spirit is another key to effective collaboration. It involves recognizing and valuing the skills of each professional, while respecting the contributions of each. Each team member brings specific expertise to the table, and the strength of a medical team lies in the diversity of these skills. It is essential to foster a climate of mutual respect, where everyone feels valued and able to express **themselves** freely. This team spirit also makes it easier to manage tensions and moments of stress, particularly in emergency **situations** where the workload is high and pressure can be intense.

Interdisciplinary collaboration is often required in complex medical situations, where several specialists must intervene for the patient's well-being. For example, in a urology department, a patient suffering from prostate cancer may require the intervention of the urologist, radiologist, pathologist, surgeon and oncologist, each bringing a different perspective to the treatment. In this type of situation, it's essential that each player is able to communicate clearly with the others, explain his or her point of view, and work together to establish a coherent overall treatment plan. Team meetings and staff meetings help to coordinate these interventions and define a common strategy for patient management.

Conflict management is an important skill in maintaining effective collaboration. In any team, differences of opinion or tensions can arise, particularly in stressful situations or when responsibilities overlap. It's important to manage these conflicts with tact and professionalism. Open, respectful dialogue is the key to resolving disagreements and finding solutions that benefit the patient first and foremost. Active listening, the ability to compromise, and respect for each other's points of view are essential qualities to prevent conflicts from hampering the quality of care.

Ongoing training also plays a crucial role in collaboration. Medical practices are constantly evolving, and it's important that team members are regularly trained in new techniques, technologies and care protocols. Caregivers, for example, can benefit from training in urinary catheter management, infection prevention or the management of post-operative patients, enabling them to improve their skills and collaborate even more effectively with other professionals. By sharing these new skills within the team, each member contributes to an overall improvement in the quality of care.

Finally, effective collaboration also implies **mutual support** between team members. Working in a medical environment can be physically and emotionally demanding. Knowing that colleagues can be counted on for support, help or even encouragement in times of difficulty is essential to maintaining a healthy, collaborative working climate. Empathy, not only towards patients, but also towards other team members, helps to build solidarity and resilience in difficult times.

    ◦   Manage logistics (emergency room preparation, close monitoring)

Managing logistics in the hospital environment, particularly in critical contexts such as emergency room preparation or close patient monitoring, is a key element in ensuring the smooth flow of care and patient safety. The nursing auxiliary plays a central role in this organization, ensuring that everything is ready and functional before patients arrive, and that equipment, medicines and materials are available and in working order. Medical logistics involves more than simply preparing equipment: it also encompasses space management, coordination with medical teams and ongoing patient monitoring to ensure fast, efficient care.

Emergency room preparation begins long before patients arrive. The orderly must ensure that the room is properly **equipped**, tidy and accessible to all members of the medical team. The first step is to check that all **resuscitation equipment** is available and ready for use. This includes **monitors** to track vital signs (heart rate, oxygen saturation, blood pressure), a **defibrillator** to manage cardiac arrest, as well as **intubation** equipment and suction devices in the event of respiratory distress. Each piece of equipment needs to be checked, particularly in terms of operation and battery charge, to ensure that it can be used without delay when needed.

Next, the caregiver must ensure that the room contains all **emergency medications**, including antidotes, vasopressors, anesthetics and sedatives. These medications should be stored in well-organized, clearly labeled **emergency carts**, so that the medical team can access them quickly and easily. Each drawer of the emergency cart should be stored systematically, with standardized organization to minimize wasted time. It is also essential to regularly check medication expiration dates to avoid any risk of shortages or delays due to expired medication.

Room layout is also a crucial factor. The space must be organized in such a way as to facilitate mobility and rapid access to equipment. It is essential to provide sufficient space around the examination table so that the different healthcare professionals can work together without getting in each other's way. The orderly ensures that everything is tidy, yet accessible, so that each member of the team can concentrate on care without having to search for the necessary equipment.

Particular attention must be paid to **sterilization** and hygiene in the emergency room. Before each procedure, surfaces must be disinfected to reduce the risk of nosocomial infections. Single-use equipment must be prepared in advance and placed on sterile trays. **Medical waste** management must also be rigorously organized. Bins for needles, syringes and other hazardous waste must be available close to the treatment area, and emptied regularly in accordance with health safety protocols.

In addition to material management, the orderly must also **anticipate the specific needs** of each emergency situation. For example, if the emergency involves trauma, **immobilizers**, **splints**, and equipment for performing **blood transfusions** or administering blood products must be provided. If the emergency is respiratory, you'll need to check that oxygen cylinders are full, and that **oxygen masks** and **nasal cannulas** are easily accessible.

This anticipation saves precious time when the emergency occurs, and ensures an immediate and adequate response to the patient's needs.

In addition to room preparation, **close patient monitoring** is another key component of logistics management. Close monitoring is often necessary for patients in critical condition, or after surgery, when their condition may change rapidly. This requires **constant vigilance** on the part of the caregiver, who must closely monitor the patient's vital signs, supervise infusions and administer prescribed treatments. The caregiver must be able to detect the first signs of deterioration in the patient's state of health, such as a drop in oxygen saturation, an abnormal acceleration in heart rate, or a change in the level of consciousness.

Regular documentation of observations is essential to ensure continuity of quality care. The caregiver must carefully record the patient's vital parameters, the treatments administered, and any clinical developments. This documentation enables the medical team to monitor the patient's progress and make informed decisions based on accurate data. Communication between teams is also a crucial factor in close monitoring. The caregiver must immediately inform the nurse or doctor of any change in the patient's condition, to enable rapid intervention if necessary.

In some cases, close monitoring also involves the use of **remote monitoring technologies**, such as portable monitors or remote monitoring devices. These technologies enable continuous monitoring of patients' vital signs, even when they are not physically present in the emergency room. Caregivers must be trained in the use of these technologies, and able to recognize alarms or alerts sent by these devices.

Finally, logistics management in an emergency context also includes **patient flow management**. The orderly must ensure that the room is ready to receive new patients after each procedure. This means quickly cleaning and reorganizing the room, restocking used equipment, and preparing the bed or examination table for the next patient. Good flow management ensures that resources are always available, and that every patient can be cared for as soon as they arrive, without unnecessary delay.

Precautions and protocol in the event of a crisis
        ◦   Ensuring patient safety

Ensuring patient safety is one of the most important responsibilities of any healthcare professional, and concerns every aspect of care, whether physical, psychological or environmental. Patient safety encompasses a series of measures designed to prevent errors, anticipate risks, and minimize incidents likely to affect the patient's health or well-being during their stay in hospital or in outpatient care. As the front line of contact with patients, the nursing auxiliary plays an essential role in implementing these safety practices on a daily basis.

The first component of patient safety is the **prevention of falls**, a frequent risk in the hospital environment, particularly among the elderly or patients weakened by surgery. To prevent these accidents, the caregiver must ensure that the patient's environment is **safe and adapted** to his or her needs. This includes checking that grab rails are correctly installed, that the bed is at the right height, and that the bed or wheelchair brakes are activated. In addition, the caregiver must be alert to the risk of clutter in the room, ensuring that no cables, bags or objects block passageways or present a tripping hazard. When a patient needs to get up or walk, it is important to provide appropriate assistance, whether in the form of direct support or the use of support devices such as walkers. Every movement must be anticipated and assisted to avoid falls and injuries.

Infection prevention is another key aspect of patient safety. In the hospital environment, patients are particularly vulnerable to nosocomial infections, especially those with invasive devices such as catheters, probes or who have just undergone surgery. Caregivers play a crucial role in enforcing strict hygiene measures to prevent these infections. This starts with rigorous compliance with **hand disinfection protocols**, before and after every patient contact, but also when handling medical devices or changing dressings. Wearing **sterile gloves**, using **hydroalcoholic solutions**, and respecting **surface cleaning protocols** are simple but essential gestures to minimize infectious risks.

Good management of medical devices is also an important part of patient safety. Urinary catheters, intravenous infusions or catheters must be handled with care and regularly monitored for any abnormalities or signs of infection. The caregiver must ensure that devices are correctly positioned, that connections are securely fastened and that there are no leaks or kinks that could impair device function. In addition, monitoring catheter or probe insertion points for signs of redness, pain or discharge enables rapid action to be taken in the event of complications.

Preventing medication errors is another essential component of patient safety. Although not directly in charge of medication administration, the nursing auxiliary is often responsible for the **preparation** and **correct identification of patients**. Before any treatment is administered, it is crucial to check the patient's identity using several criteria (surname, first name, date of birth), to avoid any confusion between patients. In case of doubt, the caregiver must always consult the nurse or doctor in charge before administering any treatment. Keeping **track of medications** and double-checking doses and dosing times also help reduce the risk of errors.

Monitoring vital parameters is a daily practice that contributes to patient safety, especially for those in critical condition or following surgery. The nursing auxiliary is often responsible for taking regular readings of temperature, blood pressure, oxygen saturation and pulse. These parameters must be accurately recorded in the patient's file, as any abnormal variation may indicate a deterioration in the patient's state of health, requiring rapid intervention by the medical team. The caregiver's role is not only to collect these data, but also to **alert immediately** in the event of any worrying sign, such as a sudden fever, a drop in blood pressure or insufficient oxygen saturation.

Effective communication with the medical team is a fundamental dimension of patient safety. Each caregiver must share all relevant information about the patient's condition, symptoms, needs and any recent changes. Good communication avoids omissions and ensures that all members of the care team have the same information to make informed decisions. For example, if a patient expresses unusual pain or symptoms, the caregiver must immediately report this information to the nurses or doctors so that they can adjust care accordingly.

Active listening and **empathy** also play a crucial role in patient safety. It is important to pay attention to patients' concerns or feelings, which can often detect the first signs of a complication. A patient expressing unusual pain, discomfort or general malaise should be taken seriously, as these signs may indicate an underlying problem. By being attentive to patients' complaints, the caregiver can act upstream to prevent the situation from worsening.

Preparing the patient before any procedure or examination is also a key moment in ensuring their safety. This includes ensuring that the patient understands what is going to happen, is fasting if necessary, or has taken their pre-operative medication as prescribed. The caregiver must ensure that the patient is properly seated, that medical devices are in place, and that he or she has been informed of the steps ahead to reduce anxiety and guarantee optimal cooperation.

Finally, ensuring patient safety also means looking after their **psychological well-being**. An anxious or stressed patient is more vulnerable to complications and less inclined to cooperate with caregivers. By taking the time to reassure patients, explain care procedures and listen to their needs, caregivers play an active role in creating a safe environment conducive to recovery.

- ∘ Protocol in the event of severe infection or postoperative complications

The **protocol for severe infection or post-operative complications** is a set of essential steps designed to identify, treat and prevent the worsening of a critical medical situation. In a hospital setting, a severe infection or post-operative complication can quickly become life-threatening if not treated quickly and effectively. The nursing auxiliary, in the front line of patient care, plays a central role in detecting early signs, communicating with the medical team and taking immediate action. Managing a postoperative infection or complication requires rigorous coordination of all healthcare professionals, and a methodical approach based on well-established protocols.

Postoperative complications can include a wide range of problems, such as infections, hemorrhage, deep vein thrombosis, organ failure, or surgical wound reopenings. **Severe infections** can manifest themselves as wound infections, urinary tract infections linked to devices such as catheters, or more serious systemic infections such as sepsis. The speed with which these complications are identified and managed is crucial to patient safety.

The **first step in the protocol** is to **identify early signs of infection or complication**. To do this, the caregiver needs to be alert to classic symptoms of infection, such as **fever** (high body temperature), **chills**, **unusual pain** or **redness** around the surgical wound, **purulent** or foul-smelling **discharge**, as well as signs of **general failure** (extreme fatigue, confusion, shortness of breath). In the case of a systemic infection, other signs such as **tachycardia**, a **drop in blood pressure** or a **reduction in diuresis** may appear, requiring immediate alerting of the medical team.

For **surgical wound** infections, daily monitoring of the surgical site is essential. The caregiver should regularly monitor the appearance of the wound, checking for signs of excessive inflammation, diffuse **redness, swelling** or **abnormal drainage**. If purulent discharge or unusual odors are detected, this may indicate infection, and a sample of secretions should be taken for microbiological analysis.

Once signs of infection or complication have been identified, **immediate communication with the medical team** is crucial. The caregiver must alert the nurse in charge or the doctor for further assessment and rapid decision-making. In this phase, **clear and precise transmission** of information is essential: the caregiver must report the symptoms observed, the duration of their onset, as well as any aggravating factors. For example, increasing pain in the vicinity of the surgical wound, accompanied by fever, must be reported in detail, as it may indicate a **deep infection** or **subcutaneous abscess**.

Immediate treatment of severe infections is usually based on the rapid administration of broad-spectrum **antibiotics**, administered intravenously to ensure rapid efficacy. The medical team draws up an **antibiotic treatment plan** based on the results of the cultures taken and the antibiogram. The orderly is responsible for monitoring the correct administration of antibiotics, respecting schedules, doses and infusion protocols. He or she is also responsible for monitoring any side effects or allergic reactions, which must be reported immediately.

For **post-operative complications** such as hemorrhage or thrombosis, more specific interventions may be required. In the event of **hemorrhage**, for example, the orderly must apply **local compression** to limit blood loss and prevent hemorrhagic shock. They must also monitor the patient's blood pressure and report any significant drop, as this could indicate decompensation. **Intravenous fluids and** sometimes **blood transfusions** may be required to restore the patient's blood volume. In some cases,

further surgery may be required to stop internal bleeding or repair a wound.

Alongside treatment of the infection or complication, **close monitoring of vital parameters** is essential. The caregiver must regularly take the patient's temperature, blood pressure and pulse, and check oxygen saturation. These data must be accurately recorded in the medical record, so that the medical team can assess the efficacy of the current treatment and adjust management if necessary. For example, if fever persists despite the administration of antibiotics, this may indicate bacterial resistance or a deeper infection that requires further investigation, such as a CT scan or ultrasound.

The management of post-operative complications is not limited to immediate medical care. It also includes **rigorous management of medical devices**. For example, a catheter-related urinary tract infection may require replacement of the catheter to eliminate the source of infection. Caregivers must ensure that devices such as urinary catheters, surgical drains or catheters are handled under strict conditions of sterility to avoid any further introduction of germs. If a catheter or drain has to be changed, the caregiver must ensure that the patient is properly informed about the procedure and is made comfortable.

Psychological support for the patient is also an important aspect of managing severe infections and postoperative complications. A patient faced with a serious infection or unexpected complication may be prey to anxiety, fear or frustration. The caregiver must demonstrate empathy, calmly explaining the treatment steps, answering the patient's questions, and providing emotional support throughout the process. Keeping patients informed about the progress of their condition and the effectiveness of treatments can help reduce anxiety and improve cooperation.

Finally, after the initial management of the infection or complication, **rigorous follow-up** must be put in place to ensure that the patient recovers properly and that complications do not recur. This includes monitoring wound healing, continuing antibiotic therapy as prescribed, and watching for any signs of relapse or new complication. In some cases, follow-up consultations with the medical team or further tests may be necessary to ensure complete resolution of the problem.

Chapter 5

The patient-caregiver relationship in urology

Psychological support for patients

　　　◦　Anxiety about urological surgery

Anxiety about urological surgery is a common phenomenon among patients, as these procedures involve intimate organs essential to vital functions such as elimination of bodily waste and reproduction. The idea of undergoing surgery of any kind can naturally arouse fear and apprehension. In urology, however, anxiety is often heightened by fear of the repercussions on quality of life, particularly with regard to urinary continence and sexual function. The caregiver, as the first point of contact in the care pathway, plays a key role in allaying these anxieties, accompanying the patient every step of the way and providing the information and support needed to alleviate this anxiety.

Preoperative anxiety in urological patients can be linked to a number of **emotional** and **physiological factors**. On the one hand, the unknown - not knowing what will happen during the operation and what the recovery period will be like - naturally gives rise to anxiety. On the other hand, urological surgery involves parts of the body that are perceived as sensitive or taboo, which increases discomfort and embarrassment. Patients wonder about the consequences of the operation on their daily lives, whether in terms of incontinence, erectile dysfunction or chronic pain. In addition, some patients may fear the anaesthetic or the length of hospital stay, while others worry about the risk of post-operative complications such as infection, bleeding or difficulty in healing.

Providing clear information is one of the best ways to reduce this anxiety. A well-informed patient is a more serene patient. In collaboration with the medical team, the caregiver can provide simple, accessible explanations of the procedure, preoperative preparations (such as the need to fast or stop certain medications), and planned postoperative care. Explaining everyone's role, from the surgeon to the anesthetist to the scrub nurse, helps to demystify the procedure and make it more understandable. It also helps to reassure the patient that common urological surgeries, such as transurethral resection of the prostate (TURP) or partial nephrectomy, are well mastered by the medical teams, and that post-operative follow-up is designed to ensure a safe recovery.

Open communication with patients is essential to address their specific concerns. Every patient is unique, and sources of stress may vary. Some are concerned about post-operative pain, others about the impact of surgery on their sexuality, or fear of loss of autonomy. By listening carefully to the patient, the caregiver can identify these sources of stress and address them proactively. For example, if a patient expresses fears about pain after surgery, it's important to explain that effective pain management strategies, including analgesics and adapted care, will be put in place to ensure his or her comfort. Similarly, if urinary incontinence is a concern, the caregiver can explain that devices such as temporary catheters are used to manage this problem, and that most patients regain good urinary control after recovery.

Empathy and presence are other powerful tools for calming anxiety. Sometimes, simply feeling listened to and supported can have a calming effect on the patient. The caregiver can take the time to be available to answer the patient's questions, reassure him or her of the competence of the care team, and provide emotional support by being attentive to the patient's reactions and state of mind. Human contact plays a fundamental role here, as it creates a relationship of trust, which is essential if patients are to feel cared for and supported. Knowing you can count on an attentive, caring team is often enough to soothe even the most nagging worries.

Relaxation techniques can also be very beneficial in reducing anxiety prior to urological surgery. For example, the caregiver can suggest deep breathing or positive visualization exercises to help the patient relax before the operation. These simple techniques, such as abdominal breathing or cardiac coherence, help to regulate the heart rate and calm the nervous system, helping to reduce tension and anxiety. Encouraging patients to focus on their breathing during stressful moments can help them to better manage their emotions and feel more in control of the situation.

What's more, **the involvement of loved ones** in the pre-operative process can play a crucial role in managing anxiety. For many patients, knowing that they are supported by family or friends can bring a sense of comfort and security. The caregiver can encourage loved ones to accompany the patient to pre-operative consultations, to be present during pre-operative preparation, or even to chat with the medical team to ensure that all questions and concerns are addressed. By involving family and friends in the process, patients feel less isolated and more supported, which can have a positive effect on their emotional state.

Once the operation is over, anxiety does not necessarily disappear. **Post-operative anxiety** may be linked to uncertainty about recovery, or the appearance of unforeseen complications. The caregiver must continue to reassure the patient after the operation, closely monitoring his or her condition and providing information on the stages of recovery. Explaining post-operative care, such as managing drains or catheters, monitoring healing and rehabilitation, helps reduce uncertainty. It's also helpful to set realistic expectations, informing the patient that certain stages of recovery, such as regaining full urinary control or managing pain, may take time. By being transparent and setting clear goals, the healthcare team helps to channel the patient's anxiety and enable him or her to focus on recovery.

○ Psychological impact of pathologies such as incontinence or cancer

The **psychological impact of pathologies** such as incontinence or cancer is profound and multifaceted. Far beyond their physical symptoms, these conditions affect patients' emotional and mental well-being, sometimes radically altering their perception of themselves, their relationship with others, and their quality of life. Incontinence, for example, affects bodily functions that are often associated with dignity and autonomy, while cancer evokes fundamental fears linked to death, serious illness and loss of control. These pathologies therefore require a holistic approach that takes into account not only medical care, but also psychological support for patients.

Urinary incontinence, whether due to surgery, age or chronic pathology, is often perceived as an affront to personal dignity. Losing control of bodily functions creates a sense of vulnerability and embarrassment in patients. Many suffer in silence, not daring to broach the subject with their loved ones or even their doctors, out of shame or fear of judgment. This silence can lead to **social isolation**, as patients fear accidents in public or the smell of urine, causing them to avoid outings, social interactions and sometimes even their professional lives. This isolation can evolve into a form of **depression** or **social anxiety**, as patients feel increasingly disconnected from the world around them, living in constant fear of an incident.

Incontinence also has an impact on **self-esteem**. Loss of urinary control can lead patients to perceive themselves as less autonomous, less capable, even "diminished". This loss of self-esteem can affect all spheres of daily life, including relationships with partners. In an intimate context, the fear of an accident or embarrassment linked to odor can lead to a **reduction in libido** and a withdrawal from sexual relations. This withdrawal can exacerbate feelings of loneliness and inadequacy, creating a vicious circle in which the pathology amplifies emotional and relational difficulties.

For a **cancer** patient, the psychological impact can be even more complex. The diagnosis of cancer is often associated with profound existential fears. The first reaction to such a diagnosis is often **shock**, followed by **emotional distress**. The prospect of a serious, and sometimes fatal, illness overwhelms the patient, who is suddenly confronted with uncertainty about the future, fear of suffering, and the idea of death. The anxiety associated with the progression of the disease, aggressive treatments such as chemotherapy or radiotherapy, and their side effects, can plunge the patient into a state of **permanent stress**.

This stress is often accompanied by a **loss of control** over one's own life. Patients may feel powerless, dispossessed of their health, and dependent on medical decisions. Frequent hospitalization, heavy treatment and surgery all contribute to this feeling of powerlessness. Cancer also imposes drastic changes in daily routine, whether due to fatigue, the side effects of treatment, or multiple medical appointments. These changes reinforce the feeling of losing one's footing and being at the mercy of the disease.

Body image is often severely affected by cancer, particularly in the case of urological cancers, which affect parts of the body involved in reproduction, sexuality and the elimination of bodily waste. Patients, especially those undergoing **prostatectomies** or **cystectomies**, may experience a **decrease in masculinity** or femininity due to the repercussions on their sexuality. The loss of erectile function in men after prostate surgery, or the need to wear a bladder bag after bladder removal, can provoke a sense of mutilation, profoundly altering the patient's relationship with his or her own body. These physical transformations reinforce the **feeling of loss of identity**, which can affect self-confidence and relationships with others.

Fear of recurrence is another psychological burden borne by cancer patients. Even after successful treatment, this fear often persists, as cancer is perceived as a permanent threat. Every minor pain or symptom can be interpreted as a sign of the disease's return, fuelling chronic stress. This anxiety, combined with regular check-ups (CT scans, blood tests, etc.), means that the patient remains constantly vigilant, unable to relax completely or resume a "normal" life.

Faced with these psychological impacts, **emotional support** is crucial for patients suffering from incontinence or cancer. Appropriate psychological support can help them cope with these emotional upheavals. It is essential to offer them a space where they can express their fears, frustrations and doubts without judgment. Healthcare professionals, particularly nursing aides, play a central role in this support by listening, answering questions and providing clear information to reduce uncertainty and anxiety.

In the case of incontinence, for example, it's important to broach the subject without taboos, explaining to the patient that solutions exist, such as absorbent devices, perineal reeducation or surgery. Knowing that the situation can be improved often helps to restore self-confidence and break the isolation. In addition, support or discussion groups can be particularly useful, enabling patients to share their experiences and feel understood.

In the case of cancer, **psychological follow-up** may include individual or group therapy sessions, as well as more targeted interventions such as stress management or relaxation. **Palliative care**, when necessary, aims not only to relieve physical pain, but also to offer psychological and spiritual support, helping patients to accept their illness and find meaning in their lives, even in the face of death.

◦   The importance of non-verbal communication

Non-verbal communication plays a fundamental role in healthcare, particularly in the relationship between caregivers and patients. It represents everything that is expressed without the use of words, whether through **body language**, **facial expressions**, **gestures** or **tone of voice**. These non-verbal signals often convey as much, if not more, information than verbal communication, as they reveal emotions, intentions and attitudes that can escape words. For caregivers, understanding and mastering non-verbal communication is essential to establishing a climate of trust, reassuring patients and improving the quality of care.

Body posture is one of the most important elements of non-verbal communication. The way a caregiver stands in the presence of a patient sends clear signals about their level of engagement, interest and empathy. An open posture, with the body facing the patient, arms relaxed and face attentive, shows that the caregiver is available and listening. Conversely, a body turned to one side, crossed arms or abrupt gestures may unintentionally suggest distance, disinterest or even aggression. The patient, often anxious or vulnerable, is highly sensitive to these signals, as he or she looks to the caregiver's attitude for clues that will make him or her feel safe and cared for. A caregiver who adopts a relaxed yet attentive posture helps the patient to feel understood and respected.

Facial expressions also play a central role in non-verbal communication. A simple smile can have an enormous impact on a patient's feelings, particularly at times of stress or anxiety. A sincere, warm smile can help dispel anxiety and build trust, as it shows that the caregiver is caring and empathetic. Conversely, a closed or distracted expression can convey a message of disinterest or impatience, even if this is not the caregiver's intention. Patients, especially those in situations of suffering or vulnerability, look to the caregiver's facial expressions for signs of understanding and reassurance. A calm, soothing face, even in tense situations, helps to calm the patient and convey the idea that the situation is under control.

Eye contact is another crucial element of non-verbal communication. Looking the patient in the eye when talking or listening is a way of showing that he or she is being taken into consideration and given full attention. Eye contact creates a bond of closeness and mutual respect, as it shows that the caregiver is fully present in the interaction. On the other hand, avoiding eye contact can be perceived as a sign of discomfort, avoidance or indifference. This can accentuate the patient's sense of isolation or abandonment, particularly at times when he or she needs reassurance or clear answers. The direct gaze, without being intrusive, should be gentle and benevolent, to show that the caregiver is open to discussion and ready to respond to the patient's questions or concerns.

Gestures and **therapeutic touch** are also powerful means of non-verbal communication. A gesture as simple as placing a hand on a patient's shoulder can bring great comfort, especially when words are insufficient to express compassion or empathy. Touch, when appropriate, can create a strong emotional bond, conveying human warmth and caring. However, it is important to respect the patient's individual and cultural limits. Some may feel uncomfortable with physical contact, so it's essential for the caregiver to read the patient's non-verbal cues to adapt his/her behavior. A reassuring gesture, such as a light touch on the arm or support during a difficult movement, can transform an interaction into a moment of shared humanity.

The **tone of voice**, although part of verbal communication, is often more influential than the words themselves. A calm, collected and reassuring tone of voice can have a calming effect on an anxious or stressed patient, far more so than the words spoken. Conversely, a brusque, authoritarian or impatient tone, even with kind words, can create distrust or anxiety in the patient. The rhythm and intensity of the voice are equally important: speaking too quickly can give the impression that the caregiver is in a hurry or unavailable, while a slow, controlled rhythm helps to create an atmosphere of calm and control. The tone of voice must therefore be adapted to the patient's emotional state, to create a harmonious and reassuring dialogue.

Proxemia, or the management of personal space, is also part of non-verbal communication and plays a crucial role in the caregiver-patient relationship. Getting too close can be perceived as an intrusion into the patient's personal space, especially in a medical environment where the patient is often already physically and emotionally vulnerable. Conversely, remaining too distant can give the impression of coldness or detachment. Finding the right distance is essential to creating a space for interaction where the patient feels respected and safe, while maintaining sufficient proximity to establish a relationship of trust.

Active listening is another aspect of non-verbal communication that has a profound impact on the quality of the caregiver-patient relationship. Active listening takes the form of simple gestures, such as nodding one's head to show that one is following the patient's speech, tilting one's body slightly towards the patient to show that one is fully attentive, or avoiding distractions such as consulting a telephone or looking away while the patient is speaking. These non-verbal signals show the patient that he or she is the focus of the caregiver's attention, reinforcing his or her sense of value and respect.

Finally, it's essential to remember that patients themselves communicate a great deal through their **own non-verbal language**. A patient who looks away, closes up in his or her posture or shows tension in his or her gestures may be expressing fear, concern or mistrust. A caregiver who is attentive to the patient's non-verbal signals is able to detect these emotions and adapt his or her response accordingly, whether through a gentler approach, reassuring words or simply an attentive presence. By observing the patient's non-verbal cues, caregivers can better understand his or her emotional needs and respond more appropriately.

Helping patients accept their illness
　　　　○　　The caregiver's role in patient information
The **caregiver's role in providing information to the patient** is essential to ensuring quality care, centered on people and respect for individual needs. Although caregivers are not directly responsible for delivering complex medical information or diagnoses, they occupy a key position in supporting patients throughout their care. By being as close as possible to the patient, the caregiver plays a crucial **interface** role between the patient and the medical team, and his or her information work contributes directly to the patient's well-being, confidence and understanding of the care he or she is receiving.

The information provided by the nursing auxiliary often begins as soon as the patient is admitted. Whether on admission to a hospital ward or prior to a medical procedure, the care assistant is often the first person to explain to the patient the **course of treatment**, **administrative steps** or **rules** to be followed within the establishment (visiting hours, hygiene instructions, etc.). This first contact is crucial, as it determines how the patient perceives his or her stay and treatment. By providing clear, comprehensible information, the caregiver helps to reduce the **anxiety** associated with the unknown, and to build a **relationship of trust**.

When preparing for a procedure, such as urological surgery for example, the nursing auxiliary must inform the patient of **pre-operative instructions** in a precise manner, adapted to the patient's condition. This may include practical information, such as fasting, not wearing jewelry, or taking an antiseptic shower. These are important details which may seem simple, but which have a direct impact on the safety of the procedure. By ensuring that the patient understands these instructions and follows them correctly, the orderly plays a key role in preparing the patient for the medical procedure.

In addition to these practical aspects, the **caregiver** also has an important role to play in **transmitting daily information** related to the care provided. They can explain to patients the basic care procedures they will be carrying out, such as taking vital parameters, grooming, changing dressings, or monitoring medical devices (catheters, probes, etc.). By taking the time to explain these gestures, the caregiver helps to establish a climate of transparency and safety. Informed in advance of what is to be done, patients feel more involved in their care and less anxious about the unknown.

For example, when inserting or changing a urinary catheter, the caregiver can explain to the patient why the catheter is needed, how it will be installed and how it will be monitored. This type of information, while seemingly routine for caregivers, is vital for the patient, enabling them to understand the process and feel more in control of the situation. By reassuring the patient that this procedure is routine and well mastered, the caregiver reduces the anxiety associated with the procedure.

The caregiver also plays a central role in **day-to-day teaching**. When the patient needs to perform specific gestures to contribute to his or her recovery, such as rehabilitation exercises, the caregiver is often responsible for explaining how to perform them correctly. This may involve, for example, perineal exercises to help regain bladder control after urological surgery. The caregiver must not only give the instructions, but also ensure that the patient has understood and is able to perform them correctly, while responding to any questions or concerns. This pedagogy is essential for the patient's autonomy and successful recovery.

Another fundamental aspect of the nursing auxiliary's role in patient information is **active listening**. When confronted with an illness or an operation, patients may be overwhelmed by questions or doubts that they don't always dare ask the doctor. By being close to the patient on a day-to-day basis, the caregiver can pick up on these questions and answer them directly when they concern practical or organizational aspects. For example, a patient may wonder how long he'll have to keep a catheter in, or whether he'll be able to walk after an operation. The caregiver, with his or her experience and proximity to the medical team, can often answer these questions or, if necessary, pass on the patient's concerns to the nurses or doctors.

Reassurance is another key aspect of the information provided by the caregiver. When faced with an anxious or uncertain patient, the caregiver's role is to provide reassuring information that helps reduce anxiety. For example, when a patient is awaiting the results of an examination or is apprehensive about an operation, the caregiver can explain the course of care to be taken and inform the patient about reasonable waiting times. Of course, the caregiver does not replace the doctor when it comes to giving results or making a diagnosis, but he or she can help **demystify certain** situations, providing clear explanations and reassuring the patient about care protocols and their effectiveness.

In addition, caregivers play an essential role in **prevention**. By informing patients about simple gestures to adopt, such as hand washing or managing medical devices at home, the caregiver contributes to infection prevention and patient safety. They can also explain the importance of certain precautions, such as respecting mobilization instructions to avoid pressure sores or post-operative complications. This educational dimension of the caregiver's role plays an active part in the health and well-being of patients, even after they have been discharged from hospital.

Finally, the nursing auxiliary also plays an important role in relaying **instructions** to the patient's family. Families often want to be involved in care, or are concerned about the aftermath of an operation. The caregiver can explain to relatives how best to support the patient, while answering practical questions about daily care, visiting hours or precautions to take at home. By providing this information, the caregiver not only helps the patient to recover more easily, but also eases the transition from hospital to home.

◦ Respecting privacy and modesty during care

Respecting privacy and modesty during care is a fundamental requirement for all healthcare professionals, and particularly for the nursing auxiliary who is in direct contact with patients on a daily basis. Every patient, whatever their state of health or situation, must feel that their body, personal space and dignity are respected. Intimacy and modesty are profound dimensions of the care relationship, and respecting them is essential not only for the psychological well-being of patients, but also for establishing a relationship of trust with them.

The first step in respecting patients' privacy is to **preserve their personal space**. In a hospital environment, the patient is often in a highly vulnerable situation, undressed or dependent on others to perform intimate gestures such as washing, changing clothes, or using medical devices. At such times, the caregiver must always bear in mind that each patient has a **different sensitivity** in terms of modesty, and that it is necessary to adapt to individual needs. When cleansing or changing dressings, for example, it's important to cover body parts not directly involved in care with a sheet or towel, to limit exposure and protect the patient's modesty.

Communication is another key element in respecting privacy. Before beginning any treatment that involves manipulation of the body or exposure of certain parts, it is essential to **inform the patient** and explain what is going to be done, why it is necessary, and how it will be carried out. By announcing each stage of care, the caregiver enables the patient to prepare mentally and physically, thus reducing anxiety and discomfort. For example, before inserting a urinary catheter or changing a surgical dressing, taking the time to explain the procedure helps the patient to feel more in control, even in a vulnerable situation. It also shows respect for the patient as an individual capable of understanding and participating in his or her care.

It's also crucial to **seek the** patient's **consent** before intervening. Although this may seem obvious in some contexts, it can sometimes be forgotten in the course of routine care. Asking the patient if they are ready, comfortable, or have any questions before proceeding with intimate care reinforces their sense of dignity and shows that the caregiver respects their body and their decisions. Even when care is unavoidable, seeking the patient's agreement is a way of recognizing his or her right to be master of his or her own body, despite medical necessity.

When providing care in the presence of others, such as in a shared room or an intensive care unit, it is imperative to **protect** the patient's **privacy** by using **screens**, curtains or asking others present to leave the room if possible. A simple gesture such as closing the door or drawing a curtain around the bed before performing intimate care shows the patient that his or her space is respected. The idea is to create a **bubble of confidentiality**, where the patient feels safe from outside scrutiny, even in an environment where privacy is difficult to maintain.

Respect for the patient's body during handling is also a crucial aspect of preserving privacy. Patient care often involves direct manipulation of the body, sometimes in particularly sensitive areas. It is essential to perform these gestures with **delicacy** and **care**, taking the time to adjust movements so that they are gentle and respectful. For example, when turning over to avoid pressure sores, or when grooming a bedridden patient, it is important to act with care, ensuring that each gesture is made in such a way as to preserve the patient's physical and emotional integrity as much as possible. This respect also involves listening to the patient's bodily signals: if they show signs of discomfort or embarrassment, it's crucial to adapt your approach.

Modesty is a concept that can vary from patient to patient, depending on their **personal history**, **culture** or **religious beliefs**. For some patients, showing a part of their body or allowing someone else to touch their privacy can be particularly difficult, even traumatic. Caregivers must therefore be attentive to these individual differences, and adapt their behavior according to each person's sensitivities. For example, some patients may prefer to be cared for by a person of the same sex, or wish to retain a degree of autonomy in intimate gestures such as grooming. Taking these preferences into account shows that the caregiver respects not only the patient's body, but also his or her **identity** and **values**.

Empathy and **benevolence** are essential qualities for respecting a patient's privacy and modesty. It's not just a question of following technical protocols, but of understanding how the patient feels about his or her vulnerability. The simple fact of recognizing that certain situations may be embarrassing or difficult for the patient, and taking this into account in his or her attitude and approach, helps to create a climate of trust. The caregiver must be attentive to signals of discomfort or unease, sometimes expressed subtly by the patient, and adjust his or her approach accordingly. Listening and patience are precious allies in making care more humane and less intrusive.

Respecting a patient's privacy and modesty also goes beyond physical care. It includes **respect for privacy** and personal information. It is important to maintain **strict confidentiality** with regard to a patient's health data, sharing this information only with the members of the healthcare team concerned, and always in compliance with the rules of professional ethics. Discussing a patient's care in his or her presence, but without including him or her in the conversation, can also be a source of discomfort or devaluation. It is therefore essential to always involve the patient in discussions concerning him or her, even when these are of a medical nature.

○ End-of-life support in urological palliative care

Urological palliative care at **the end of life** is a profoundly human and delicate stage, where the aim is no longer to cure, but to relieve pain, offer comfort, and respect the patient's dignity until his or her last moments. This care is focused on improving quality of life - physical, psychological and emotional - while taking into account the specific needs of patients suffering from advanced urological pathologies, such as prostate or bladder cancer, or end-stage renal failure. The caregiver plays a central role in this support, often being the person closest to the patient, providing technical care, psychological support and a reassuring presence.

Palliative care support begins with comprehensive management of **pain** and physical symptoms. In urological pathologies, this often includes management of symptoms such as **incontinence, recurrent urinary tract infections**, **urinary retention**, or pain associated with bone metastases in prostate cancer. Caregivers play a key role in monitoring symptoms and administering treatments to relieve them. He or she must ensure that devices such as urinary catheters or catheters are correctly positioned and function properly, taking care that these devices do not add extra pain or discomfort. The patient's physical comfort is the priority, and the caregiver must adjust care according to individual needs, in collaboration with the medical team.

Pain relief in palliative care often relies on drug treatments such as high-level analgesics (morphine and other opioids). Although not directly responsible for prescribing these drugs, the caregiver must monitor their effectiveness, report any signs of discomfort or unrelieved pain, and adjust patient positions to prevent pressure points or pressure sores. He or she is also responsible for hygiene and infection prevention, performing skin care and intimate hygiene with the utmost gentleness, in order to preserve the patient's dignity while avoiding further complications.

Support at the end of life is not limited to the physical dimension. It also includes **psychological and emotional** support. Patients at the end of life may feel anguish, sadness, anger or profound loneliness as they approach death. The caregiver is often a reassuring and comforting presence at these moments, providing attentive, non-judgmental listening. Sometimes it's simply a matter of being there, holding the patient's hand, offering a soothing presence. The end of life is a time of great vulnerability, and the caregiver's caring attitude helps the patient feel understood, heard and supported.

Urological palliative care can also involve delicate situations relating to **modesty** and **intimacy**. Care such as the management of incontinence or urinary catheters touches on very personal aspects of the patient's body. Caregivers must take extra care to respect the patient's modesty and intimacy, taking care to cover the patient as much as possible, explaining each gesture with delicacy, and ensuring that this care is carried out in a private and respectful environment. Maintaining the patient's dignity until his or her last moments is a priority, as it helps preserve self-esteem and a sense of control over the body, even in this terminal phase.

Family support is also an integral part of end-of-life care. The patient's loved ones are often faced with distress, questions about their loved one's suffering, and the anticipation of bereavement.

Through their experience and humanity, caregivers act as mediators between the nursing team and families. They can provide simple information on ongoing care, reassure loved ones that everything is being done to ensure the patient's comfort, and offer empathetic listening. The emotional support they provide to families reduces their anxiety, helps them to better understand the situation, and sometimes guides them in the gradual acceptance of the impending loss.

In palliative care, it is also important to respect the **patient's wishes**. Some patients may wish to limit certain invasive treatments, or request special arrangements for their final moments. The caregiver must respect these choices, ensuring that the patient's wishes are heard and followed, through advance directives or discussions with the care team. This may include decisions about limiting medical interventions, adapting care to offer greater comfort, or even spiritual and religious choices that need to be honored.

Time spent with a patient at the end of life is invaluable. Unlike conventional medical care, where time is often limited, palliative care leaves room for human accompaniment, where time is no longer focused solely on technical acts, but on listening, being present and sharing. Sometimes, a patient at the end of life no longer has the words to express his or her needs, but their suffering or discomfort can be felt through non-verbal signals that the caregiver, with his or her experience and attention, is able to pick up on. It's a question of understanding silences, perceiving gestures or glances that speak volumes about the patient's state of mind.

End-of-life care in a urological palliative care setting therefore requires not only technical know-how, but above all **interpersonal skills**. The caregiver is a **pillar of benevolence** at these moments, providing unfailing support, personalized accompaniment and attention to every detail. He or she is a guardian of the patient's dignity and humanity, ensuring that, even in his or her final moments, the patient is treated with the respect he or she deserves. This end-of-life care is a profoundly humanistic act, where technique and compassion come together to enable the patient to live his or her last moments as serenely as possible.

Managing relationships with loved ones
        ◦   Involving family members in daily care

Involving loved ones in day-to-day care is a fundamental aspect of patient care, particularly when the patient is faced with a chronic illness, surgery or dependency. The presence and support of loved ones is not only emotionally beneficial, they can also play an active role in daily care, helping to improve the patient's quality of life and lighten the workload of care teams. In this dynamic, the caregiver occupies a key position, acting as an intermediary between the medical team, the patient and his or her loved ones, facilitating their integration into the care process.

The **emotional aspect** of involving loved ones is crucial. Their presence provides the patient with a sense of security, comfort and love, which can considerably reduce anxiety and distress, especially at times when the patient feels vulnerable or helpless. Loved ones are often the people the patient trusts most, and this trust manifests itself in emotional soothing when they are involved in care. Whether it's a simple gesture such as accompanying the patient to the toilet, helping him/her to settle comfortably in bed, or being present at difficult moments, their support is essential to the patient's psychological equilibrium.

However, the involvement of loved ones is not limited to a simple emotional presence. They can be **actively involved** in more hands-on care, under the supervision and guidance of healthcare professionals. The caregiver plays a crucial role in **training** and **guiding relatives** to carry out certain tasks, according to the patient's needs. For example, when caring for a urological pathology, a relative can be trained to help the patient manipulate a urinary catheter or monitor a **catheter**, under the caregiver's instructions, ensuring that care continues safely outside the times when medical staff are available.

Training for loved ones must be adapted to their level of understanding and comfort with medical procedures. Some relatives may be at ease with the technical aspects of care, while others may be reluctant or fearful of the responsibility of intervening in the bodily care of their loved one. The caregiver must be attentive to these reactions, offering personalized support that respects the learning pace and preferences of each individual. This may involve teaching simple gestures, such as how to reposition a bedridden patient to avoid pressure sores, or explaining how to watch for signs of infection around a surgical wound or medical device.

Involving family and friends in care also **helps to facilitate the return home** and continuity of care after hospitalization. When a patient leaves hospital, he or she may still need daily care, such as managing medication, changing dressings or performing rehabilitation tasks. The caregiver, in collaboration with the nurses, must prepare relatives for these tasks before the patient leaves. This includes not only learning the techniques, but also understanding the **warning signs** that could indicate a complication (fever, pain, redness, swelling) and necessitate a return to hospital. By training relatives, the caregiver not only makes them more competent, but also more confident in their ability to handle these situations, reducing the stress and anxiety associated with caring for a patient at home.

Accompanying loved ones in their care must also include a **human** and empathetic **dimension**. For many people, watching a loved one suffer or depending on daily support can be emotionally draining. They may feel helpless, sad or even frustrated by the illness. The caregiver's role is one of **moral support**, listening to the concerns of loved ones, recognizing the difficulty of their role, and reassuring them that they are not alone in this process. Offering them moments of exchange and experience-sharing can help them better understand the situation and accept the challenges of caregiving.

Another important aspect of family and friends' involvement is **care coordination**. By being involved in day-to-day care, relatives can also become crucial information relays between the patient and the medical team. They are often the first to notice changes in the patient's state of health, signs of deterioration, or improvements. The caregiver must encourage this dialogue, regularly asking relatives to share their observations, and explaining which elements need to be monitored. This dialogue is invaluable for adjusting care and ensuring that the patient receives the necessary attention at the right time.

Involving family and friends does not mean they have to carry the burden of care alone. It's important to remind them that the medical team is always there to **support** and **take over** when necessary. The caregiver must ensure that relatives do not feel overwhelmed by their new responsibilities, and that they know they can ask for help or advice at any time. It is also essential to ensure that relatives have time to rest, and that they can **preserve their own equilibrium**. Caring for a patient at home, especially one at the end of life or suffering from a debilitating chronic illness, can be physically and emotionally exhausting. Caregivers can point them in the direction of respite solutions, such as home help services or temporary stays in care facilities, so that they can recharge their batteries guilt-free.

The involvement of loved ones in care also extends to **taking into account the wishes of** the patient and his or her family. Some patients, especially at the end of life, may have specific wishes concerning the care they do or do not wish to receive. The caregiver must ensure that these wishes are respected and communicated to the care team. This includes the way in which care is provided, the choice to remain at home or in an institution, and any spiritual or religious aspects that may be important to the patient and family. Respecting these wishes enhances the patient's dignity, and allows relatives to feel more involved and in agreement with the decisions made.

○ Appropriate communication with the family

Appropriate communication with the family is an essential component of caregivers' work, particularly in situations where the patient is seriously ill, convalescing or in palliative care. The patient's family, be they relatives, friends or primary carers, often plays a central role in support, decision-making and follow-up care. For the caregiver, it is crucial to develop clear, empathetic and family-friendly communication, as this not only helps to reassure relatives, but also to create an environment of trust and cooperation, to the benefit of the patient.

The first step in **appropriate communication** with the family is to establish a relationship based on **transparency** and **active listening**. The patient's loved ones are often worried, going through periods of uncertainty, anxiety and stress. The caregiver must therefore ensure that they are listened to, paying attention to their concerns, questions and needs. This means offering them a space where they can freely express their fears and questions. By responding accurately and honestly, the caregiver helps to ease tensions and build trust. It is essential to avoid complex medical jargon, which can reinforce misunderstandings, and to favor clear, accessible language, so that the family can fully understand the patient's state of health and the care provided.

Empathy is a crucial dimension of communication with families. Every family reacts differently to the illness or deteriorating health of a loved one. Some may be very worried, asking many questions, while others may be more silent or resigned. The caregiver must be **sensitive** to these varied reactions, adapting his or her approach according to the family's emotional state. It's important to recognize the suffering or anxiety that loved ones are going through, and to show them that they are not alone in this ordeal. A comforting word, attention to their needs or a caring

120

presence can make a big difference, no matter how difficult the situation.

Caregivers must also ensure that they **provide regular information** on the patient's condition. Families often want to be kept informed of their loved one's progress, especially when the patient is in a critical or end-of-life situation. In collaboration with the medical team, the caregiver can offer updates on current care, explain upcoming procedures or answer questions about treatments being administered. This transparency helps families better understand what's going on, prepare for possible changes and feel more involved in the care process. However, it is important to respect the respective roles: complex medical information should be relayed by the doctor, while the caregiver can supplement this information with practical explanations or advice on day-to-day care management.

In some cases, the family may have to make **difficult decisions** about care, particularly in palliative or end-of-life care. The caregiver, although not in charge of medical decisions, can offer invaluable support by being a **sympathetic interlocutor** for the family. They can help clarify certain practical aspects of care, answer questions about the implications of certain decisions (for example, stopping invasive treatments), or simply offer an attentive ear. At such times, the caregiver can also refer the family to resources, such as teams of psychologists or support services, to help them through this difficult period.

Appropriate communication with the family must also take into account **cultural** or religious **preferences and sensitivities**. Each family has its own values and beliefs, which influence the way it perceives illness, death or medical care. The caregiver must be attentive to these particularities, respecting the wishes expressed by the family or the patient concerning rituals, religious practices or end-of-life decisions. It is important not to impose a standardized medical point of view, but to seek to understand and integrate the family's specific needs, ensuring that these are taken into account in the care provided.

One of the challenges of communicating with the family is knowing how to **manage** any **tensions or conflicts** that may arise. Moments of illness or distress can exacerbate family tensions, and it is not uncommon for disagreements to arise over decisions to be made for the patient. The caregiver, in this context, must remain neutral and professional, while being attentive to these dynamics. He or she can help calm tensions by promoting dialogue and encouraging calm discussion between family members and the medical team. Sometimes, simply clarifying care or treatment options can reduce misunderstandings and ease conflicts.

Appropriate **non-verbal communication** is also very important when interacting with the family. Simple gestures, such as a smile, a kind look or a discreet but available presence, can help to reassure the family, especially when it is difficult to find the right words. The caregiver must be **present** and **attentive**, even at times when verbal exchanges are limited. Silent but respectful accompaniment can offer great comfort, especially when the family is going through moments of uncertainty or sadness.

Finally, the caregiver can be an **invaluable** ally in supporting families after discharge from hospital or the end of care. When the patient returns home or is transferred to an institution, the family may feel helpless when it comes to continuing care at home or managing day-to-day life. By providing clear explanations of the care to be carried out at home, giving practical advice or referring the family to home help services, the caregiver helps to reassure relatives and make them more autonomous in caring for the patient.

Chapter 6

Technological tools and innovations in urology

Cutting-edge diagnostic and treatment technologies
  ◦   CT scan, MRI, urological ultrasound
Medical imaging examinations such as **CT**, **MRI** and **urological ultrasound** are essential tools in the diagnosis and management of urological diseases. These techniques provide precise, detailed images of the organs of the urinary system, including the kidneys, bladder, ureters and prostate, as well as certain surrounding structures. Each of these methods has its own specific features, advantages and indications, enabling doctors to assess the state of health of the organs concerned, detect abnormalities and plan appropriate treatments. In this context, the nursing auxiliary plays a central role, accompanying patients throughout the process, reassuring them and preparing them before the examinations.

CT scanning is an imaging technique that uses X-rays to produce cross-sectional images of the body. This type of examination is often used in urology to diagnose and evaluate conditions such as **kidney stones**, kidney or bladder **tumors**, or to detect structural abnormalities in the urinary tract. CT scans are particularly effective in visualizing the body's internal structures with great precision, especially when combined with the injection of a contrast medium, which enables blood vessels and tissues to be better visualized.

The role of the caregiver is crucial in preparing the patient for a **urological scan**. He or she must explain the examination to the patient, reassuring him or her that it is painless and relatively quick. If a contrast medium is used, the caregiver must check for any **contraindications**, such as allergies to iodine or kidney problems, and ensure that the patient is fasting if required. The patient is then placed comfortably on the scanner table, and the caregiver ensures that he or she is correctly positioned to guarantee quality images. Once the examination has begun, it is essential to remind the patient to remain still to avoid artifacts on the images, while remaining available to answer any questions or concerns.

MRI (Magnetic Resonance Imaging) is another advanced imaging technique that uses magnetic fields and radio waves to create highly detailed images of internal organs. In urology, MRI is particularly useful for evaluating **prostate** and **kidney tumors**, or for detecting complex abnormalities of the urinary tract. MRI has the advantage of providing highly accurate images of soft tissues, making it easier to differentiate benign from malignant tumors, and to assess the extent of cancer, particularly in the case of the prostate.

However, MRI is a longer and more demanding examination than CT scanning, due to the time required to acquire images and the significant noise generated by the machine. This is why patient preparation and support are essential. The caregiver must prepare the patient by checking that there are no contraindications, such as the presence of pacemakers, metal prostheses or metallic foreign bodies in the body. They must also ensure that the patient is comfortable with the idea of remaining motionless in a narrow tunnel for several minutes. Some patients suffer from **claustrophobia**, so it's important to reassure them before the examination, explaining that they will be able to communicate with the technician during the MRI via an intercom system. The caregiver plays a calming role here, listening to the patient and making sure that everything is done to ensure that the examination takes place in the best possible conditions.

Urological ultrasound is a more common and simpler imaging method, using **ultrasound** to visualize the organs of the urinary system. It's a non-invasive, painless examination that generally requires no special preparation, and is often used as a first-line procedure to explore symptoms such as abdominal pain, urinary disorders or the detection of masses. In urology, ultrasound is used to examine the **kidneys**, **bladder** and **prostate** in men. Ultrasound is particularly useful for detecting kidney stones, tumors or cysts, and for assessing prostate size, especially in cases of benign prostatic hyperplasia (BPH).

125

One of the advantages of ultrasound is that it can be carried out quickly and in conditions that are relatively comfortable for the patient. The caregiver prepares the patient by explaining the procedure and ensuring that he or she has drunk enough water to fill the bladder, if necessary for the ultrasound. The assistant then helps the patient to settle on the examination table, ensuring that he or she is well positioned to allow the doctor or technician to perform the ultrasound in the best possible conditions. During the examination, the caregiver ensures the patient's comfort and remains close by to respond to his or her needs.

In some cases, a **transrectal ultrasound** may be necessary to obtain more precise images of the prostate. This examination can be more uncomfortable for the patient, as it involves inserting a probe into the rectum. Here again, the caregiver plays a crucial role in **reassuring the patient**, explaining that the discomfort is temporary and that the examination provides precise information essential for diagnosis.

On the whole, these imaging techniques - CT scan, MRI and ultrasound - are complementary, providing an accurate overview of urological pathologies. **CT** is often preferred for its speed and ability to detect abnormalities such as stones or tumors, while **MRI** is used for more in-depth exploration of soft tissues, particularly in cases of cancer. **Ultrasound**, on the other hand, is an easy-to-perform, non-invasive first-line examination that provides rapid information on the state of the organs of the urinary system.

The caregiver's role in this context is not only to prepare the patient technically for the examinations, but also to support them emotionally, by answering their questions and reassuring them throughout the process. Thanks to this caring approach, the caregiver helps to **reduce** patients' **anxiety** in the face of these sometimes impressive examinations, and to ensure that everything runs smoothly to obtain the results needed for diagnosis and treatment.

○ Surgical robotics and minimally invasive procedures

Surgical robotics and **minimally invasive procedures** are revolutionizing modern surgery, particularly in urology. These technological advances enable surgeons to perform complex procedures with unrivalled precision, while minimizing trauma to the patient. Thanks to sophisticated tools such as the **Da Vinci surgical system**, robotics offer greater control over surgical gestures, three-dimensional visualization of tissues, and millimetric precision in the execution of procedures. These innovations have profoundly transformed the way certain urological pathologies, such as prostate cancer, kidney stones or renal tumours, are managed, improving clinical outcomes and reducing post-operative complications.

Minimally invasive procedures are distinguished from traditional surgery by their less aggressive approach. Rather than opening the abdominal cavity wide, as in conventional open surgery, minimally invasive techniques use small incisions through which specialized instruments are inserted. In urology, this can include procedures such as **radical prostatectomy** (removal of the prostate), **partial nephrectomy** (partial removal of the kidney), or **cystectomy** (removal of the bladder), performed with the aid of a surgical robot or laparoscopy. The aim of these procedures is to minimize trauma to the patient, by reducing the size of incisions and limiting disruption to surrounding tissue.

The **Da Vinci system**, the most widely used surgical robot in the world, is a perfect example of the progress made by robotics in surgery. The robot consists of several articulated arms, operated by the surgeon from a console. The surgeon controls each of these arms with unrivalled precision, thanks to an interface that reproduces his or her movements in real time, but on a miniaturized scale. One of the arms holds a camera, providing a three-dimensional, high-definition view of the inside of the body, while the other handles the surgical instruments. The **3D vision provided by** the system, combined with the **stability of the**

127

robotic instruments, enables the surgeon to work with far greater precision than would be possible with manual surgery alone. This is particularly important for delicate procedures, such as preserving the nerves responsible for urinary continence or erectile function during prostatectomy.

The benefits of surgical robotics are numerous, for patients and surgeons alike. For the patient, these minimally invasive techniques generally mean smaller incisions, reducing intraoperative bleeding, lowering the risk of infection and accelerating healing. Post-operative pain is also less intense, enabling **faster recovery** and an earlier return to daily activities. For example, in the case of **robot-assisted prostatectomy**, hospitalization time is often reduced to a few days, compared with a week or more for open surgery. In addition, functional results are often better, with faster recovery of continence and sexual function, as robotics enable more precise dissection of nerve and vascular structures.

For surgeons, the use of robotics offers significantly improved **working comfort**. Unlike open surgery, which can be physically demanding, requiring long hours on their feet, the surgeon using the robot sits at a console, manipulating instruments in an ergonomic position. This reduces fatigue during long, complex procedures. What's more, robotic instruments offer **better dexterity** than human hands, with finer, more precise movements, eliminating natural tremors. This precision is particularly beneficial in delicate surgeries, where the margin for error is minimal, such as a **partial nephrectomy** to remove a renal tumor while preserving the rest of the kidney.

In addition to robotics, **minimally invasive procedures** in urology also include **endoscopic surgery** and **percutaneous** techniques. **Ureteroscopy**, for example, is a technique whereby an endoscope is inserted into the urinary tract, via the urethra, to treat kidney stones or bladder tumours. This endoscopic approach eliminates the need for external incisions, considerably reducing recovery time and wound complications. Similarly, **percutaneous**

128

lithotripsy, a technique used to break up kidney stones, is performed through a small incision in the skin, allowing direct access to the kidney to treat the stones, without the need for open surgery.

Minimally invasive and robotic techniques have profoundly changed the **way** urology patients are **cared for**. They not only improve functional results, but also **reduce** long-term **complications** such as postoperative infections, bleeding and hernias. Shorter recovery times mean shorter hospital stays, a quicker return to normal life and lower costs for the healthcare system.

The role of the **caregiver** in this context is central. Before the operation, the caregiver is often the first point of contact to reassure the patient, explain the procedure and check that he or she has understood the pre-operative instructions, such as the need to fast. During the procedure, the orderly works with the surgical team to ensure that all the necessary equipment is in place and that the patient is correctly positioned for the robotic or laparoscopic operation. After the operation, the orderly plays a key role in **post-operative monitoring**, helping with pain management, monitoring the patient's vital signs and ensuring that convalescence takes place in the best possible conditions.

Finally, the caregiver plays an active role in **educating the patient** and his or her family after the operation. It's important that the patient understands how to care for his or her surgical wounds, the warning signs to watch out for, such as fever or abnormal bleeding, and the recommendations for gradually resuming physical activities. The caregiver therefore plays a fundamental role in the **transition to home**, offering practical advice and answering the patient's questions about his or her convalescence.

The impact of new technologies on the caregiver's work
- ◦ Technological equipment management (probes, monitoring devices)

The **management of technological equipment**, such as **probes** and **monitoring devices**, is an essential component of medical care, particularly in urology. This equipment enables continuous monitoring of the patient's condition, the performance of certain physiological functions or the administration of treatments. Their effective use depends not only on technological precision, but also on the ability of caregivers to handle and maintain them correctly, and to prevent complications associated with their use. The caregiver plays a central role in this management, ensuring that the devices function correctly, that the patient is safe, and that vital information is transmitted to the medical team.

Catheters are among the most frequently used items of equipment in a urology department. The **urinary catheter**, for example, is a device inserted into the urethra to drain urine directly from the bladder. It is commonly used in situations where the patient is unable to urinate normally, whether due to an obstruction, after surgery, or as a result of pathology. Urinary catheter management requires **careful monitoring** to prevent complications such as urinary tract infections or catheter blockage.

The caregiver, in the front line, must ensure that the catheter is correctly positioned and that the drainage system functions smoothly. This means regularly checking that the catheter is not twisted or obstructed, and that the urine collection bag is emptied at regular intervals to avoid overloading. The caregiver should also observe **urine quality** (color, clarity and odor), as this can be an early indicator of infection or complication. For example, if the urine becomes cloudy or smells foul, this may suggest a urinary tract infection. These observations should be reported immediately to the nurse or doctor, so that prompt action can be taken.

One of the most critical aspects of catheter management is **infection prevention**. The insertion of a urinary catheter, although commonplace, represents a potential route of entry for bacteria, exposing the patient to the risk of nosocomial infection. Caregivers must therefore scrupulously observe **aseptic** protocols when handling the catheter. This includes washing hands, wearing sterile gloves and disinfecting the catheter insertion area. It is also essential to **change the catheter regularly**, in line with medical recommendations, to limit the risk of bacterial colonization. When replacing the catheter, the caregiver must explain the process to the patient, ensuring that he or she is well informed and reassured, as this procedure can be a source of discomfort.

Monitoring devices also play a major role in tracking a patient's state of health. They enable real-time monitoring of vital parameters such as heart rate, oxygen saturation (SpO2), blood pressure and body temperature. In a urological context, these devices are often used after surgery or when managing a patient in critical condition. For example, after prostatectomy or nephrectomy, vital signs monitoring is essential for early detection of post-operative complications such as hemorrhage or infection.

The caregiver is responsible for **setting up** and **monitoring** these devices. He/she must ensure that the heart monitor electrodes are correctly positioned, that the oxygen saturation sensor is correctly attached to the patient's finger, and that the blood pressure cuff is in place for reliable measurements. In the event of a device malfunction (false alarm, incorrectly positioned sensor), the caregiver must intervene quickly to resolve the problem, taking care not to interrupt continuous monitoring of the patient. Good management of these devices requires constant vigilance and the ability to interpret the data provided, in order to quickly identify abnormal variations and report them to the medical team.

In addition to monitoring vital parameters, the caregiver must also be attentive to the **patient's reactions**. Some devices, although not very invasive, can be uncomfortable for patients. For example, the prolonged wearing of an automatic blood pressure cuff can cause discomfort, just as a saturation sensor can cause skin irritation if held in place for too long. The caregiver must therefore ensure the patient's **well-being** by adjusting devices in such a way as to minimize discomfort, while guaranteeing their effectiveness.

Vigilance and responsiveness are essential skills in the management of monitoring systems. Vital signs monitor alarms are warning signals that must be interpreted quickly. A sudden drop in oxygen saturation, a fall in blood pressure or an acceleration in heart rate may indicate a deterioration in the patient's condition, requiring immediate intervention. The orderly, in the front line when faced with these alarms, must assess the situation quickly, check whether the problem is due to a technical malfunction or a genuine medical complication, and alert the nurse or doctor accordingly.

In addition to monitoring devices and catheters, other technological equipment such as **infusion pumps** or **patient-controlled analgesia (PCA) pumps** are commonly used in hospitals. Infusion pumps enable fluids, nutrients or medications to be administered in a controlled manner. The caregiver must ensure that infusions are correctly programmed, that tubing is not blocked or kinked, and that the flow rate is respected. PCA pumps, used for pain relief, allow the patient to self-administer a controlled dose of analgesic at the touch of a button. Here again, the caregiver must monitor the patient's use of the pump, ensuring that the device is working properly and that the patient understands how it works. He or she must also monitor potential side effects associated with PCA use, such as drowsiness or respiratory depression, and report any abnormal signs to the medical team.

Finally, equipment maintenance is an essential aspect of technological device management. The caregiver must ensure that each device is **disinfected** after use, in accordance with hygiene protocols, to prevent the spread of infection. Probes, catheters, monitoring sensors and tubing must be carefully handled and cleaned, or discarded if they are single-use. Particular attention must be paid to the **sterility of** equipment, especially when handling urinary catheters and infusions, to minimize the risk of introducing germs into the patient's body.

 ◦   Assist the surgical team in the use of robots

Assisting the surgical team when using **surgical robots** is an essential and demanding responsibility, particularly in complex procedures where technological precision is paramount. The rise of **surgical robotics**, notably with systems such as the **Da Vinci**, has transformed the way certain operations are performed, especially in urology, enabling surgeons to work with greater precision while minimizing trauma to the patient. The assistance of nurses and paramedical staff in this context is essential to ensure that operations run smoothly, whether before, during or after the operation.

In the first instance, even before the operation, the orderly plays an important role in **preparing the operating room** and the equipment. When surgical robots are used, equipment management becomes even more complex than for traditional surgery, requiring **meticulous set-up** of robotic arms, instruments and control consoles. The caregiver must ensure that all the equipment required for the procedure is correctly arranged, disinfected and functional. The robot arms, which can be equipped with a variety of surgical tools, must be carefully positioned around the operating table, taking into account the access required by the surgeon and other team members.

At the same time, the caregiver **prepares the patient** for the robotic procedure. They ensure that the patient is correctly positioned on the operating table, according to the surgeon's instructions. In robotics, patient positioning is particularly important, as robotic instruments require **precise access** to the areas to be operated on. The caregiver therefore ensures that the patient is well immobilized, using positioning cushions or straps, to guarantee that he/she will not move during the operation. They also ensure that the patient's skin is disinfected and that sterile drapes are applied in compliance with hygiene protocols, thus limiting the risk of infection.

Once the robot is in place and the patient is ready, the caregiver works with the surgical team to ensure **continuous assistance** throughout the procedure. Although the surgeon controls the robotic arms from a console located a few meters from the operating table, it is essential to have a team present with the patient to manage the non-robotic aspects of the procedure. The orderly often assists the operating room nurse or assistant surgeon by providing additional instruments, adjusting the patient's position if necessary, or helping to manage surgical fluids.

One of the caregiver's crucial roles is to **monitor the patient** during the procedure. Indeed, although the surgeon is focused on the control screen, it is vital that someone is in the immediate vicinity of the patient to monitor vital signs and ensure that everything is going well physically. This includes managing monitoring devices such as heart rate, blood pressure and oxygen saturation monitors. The caregiver must be able to quickly detect any signs of deterioration in the patient's condition and alert the team to any problems, ensuring maximum safety throughout the procedure.

The caregiver also plays a crucial role in **managing the robotic equipment** during the operation. Although the surgeon is in full control of the robot's movements, it may be necessary to adjust or reposition the robotic arms during the operation to allow better access to certain areas of the body. The orderly, under the supervision of the surgeon or OR nurse, may be required to make these adjustments, while ensuring that the sterility of the operating field is maintained. The caregiver's responsiveness and precision at these moments are essential to ensure the smooth running of the operation.

At the end of the operation, the caregiver is involved in the **immediate post-operative management of** the patient. After removal of the robotic instruments and arms, the caregiver helps reposition the patient on the table, ready for transfer to the recovery room. He also ensures that the small incisions made for robotic arm access are properly sutured, and that the patient is cleaned and covered to prevent hypothermia, a frequent concern after a long operation.

The management of post-operative equipment is also crucial. The nursing auxiliary is involved in **disinfecting** and **preparing the robot** for future operations. The robotic instruments used are often complex and costly, requiring meticulous maintenance to ensure their long-term operability. The caregiver, in collaboration with the technical team, ensures that robotic arms and instruments are properly cleaned, sterilized and reassembled if necessary.

In addition to the technical aspects, the caregiver has an important role to play in **communicating with the patient** before and after the operation. Before the operation, the use of robotics can raise questions and concerns in the patient. It is essential that the caregiver is able to provide clear and reassuring explanations of how the procedure will be carried out. Although the surgeon provides the detailed information, the caregiver can play a supportive role by explaining the practical aspects of using the robots and by answering the patient's questions with empathy. After the operation, the caregiver continues to support the patient by explaining post-operative care, such as managing incisions or monitoring for signs of complications.

The nursing auxiliary also acts as a **liaison** between the patient and the medical team after the operation. They ensure that the patient is properly settled in the recovery room, and that vital parameters are closely monitored. If necessary, the caregiver can answer questions from the patient or relatives, explaining how the operation went and what the next steps in recovery will be. This human support is particularly important in surgery involving sophisticated technologies such as robotics, as the patient may feel impressed by the technological aspect of the operation.

Ongoing training and adaptation to innovation
   ◦   Importance of continuing education

The **importance of continuing education** for healthcare professionals, and particularly for nursing assistants, cannot be overstated. In a constantly evolving field, where technological advances, new medical practices and scientific discoveries regularly transform standards of care, continuing education is essential to ensure optimal patient care. It enables caregivers to keep abreast of the latest techniques, enhance their practical skills and enrich their theoretical knowledge. For the caregiver, continuing education is an essential tool for maintaining a high level of competence, adapting to the new demands of the profession, and offering quality care, while contributing to his or her own professional and personal development.

Healthcare is a dynamic field, with constant advances in treatments, technologies and care protocols. The emergence of new diseases, discoveries about existing pathologies or advances in surgical procedures mean that caregivers are constantly updating their knowledge. For example, the introduction of **surgical robotics** and **minimally invasive procedures** has profoundly altered the way operations are performed in urology and other specialties. A nursing assistant working in a surgical department needs to be trained in these technologies to be able to assist the medical team effectively and understand the implications for post-operative patient care.

Patient safety is directly linked to the competence of caregivers, and ongoing training helps to reduce the risk of errors, improve practices and ensure that care always complies with the latest standards. For example, in the field of nosocomial infection prevention, new recommendations may be published regularly, whether in terms of hand hygiene, management of medical devices (probes, catheters) or wound care. By attending regular training courses, orderlies can ensure that they apply these protocols to the letter, minimizing risks to patients.

In addition, **ongoing training** enables us to learn how to manage new or exceptional situations. For example, with the emergence of new epidemics or pandemics, such as COVID-19, caregivers had to adapt their practices overnight. Specific training in personal protection protocols, management of patients with contagious diseases and disinfection of care areas was essential to protect both patients and care staff. Similarly, training in palliative care techniques and pain management is essential to better support patients at the end of life, particularly in oncology and palliative care departments.

In addition to the technical aspects, continuing training also helps to strengthen the **interpersonal skills** and human aspects of care. Caregivers are often on the front line in dealing with patients and their families. Training in **communicating with patients** can be very helpful in better understanding their needs and expectations, especially in situations of emotional fragility or distress. Learning to listen more effectively, to respond with empathy, or to manage situations of conflict or tension with families is just as important as mastering technical gestures. These **cross-disciplinary** skills are essential if we are to offer holistic care, focused not just on the disease, but on the whole person.

Ongoing training also enables **specific skills** to be **developed** as the role of the nursing auxiliary evolves in certain departments. For example, with the introduction of advanced technologies such as remote monitoring devices, caregivers need to learn how to use these tools to monitor patients' vital parameters. Similarly, in the field of telemedicine, which has developed strongly in recent years, caregivers may need to participate in the management of remote consultations. In these contexts, ongoing training is essential to integrate these new practices into everyday care.

One of the major advantages of continuing training is that it contributes to the **professional development of** care assistants. By following specialized training courses, they can broaden their skills, take on new responsibilities or consider career development. For example, an orderly who specializes in palliative care or robotic surgery assistance can become an expert in these fields, and be recognized as a valuable resource for the medical team. What's more, some training courses enable the acquisition of skills that lead to gateways to other care professions, such as nursing or health management.

On a personal level, continuing education also helps to **maintain motivation** and commitment to one's work. It gives caregivers the opportunity to feel valued and to enrich their daily practice. The feeling of progressing, of learning new things and of better mastering one's profession is a powerful factor in job satisfaction. This helps to combat **routine** and avoid **burnout**, which can sometimes occur in professions as emotionally and physically demanding as nursing care.

Today, there is a wide range of training options available. **Face-to-face training sessions**, organized in hospitals or training centers, enable orderlies to learn in a practical way, by exchanging ideas with trainers and colleagues. **Online training** has also become increasingly popular, offering invaluable flexibility, especially for caregivers who have to manage irregular schedules. These online modules provide autonomous access to up-to-date content, accompanied by tutorials, videos and quizzes to validate knowledge. These systems also offer the opportunity to follow training courses on highly specialized topics, which would not always be available locally.

Finally, ongoing training plays a key role in **adapting to new** healthcare **regulations** and standards. Legal requirements and public health policies evolve regularly, and it's essential that caregivers keep abreast of new legislation, patient rights, safety guidelines and regulations relating to the confidentiality of medical data. By attending regular training courses, caregivers can ensure that they comply with these standards and work within a secure legal framework, both for themselves and for patients.

In short, **continuous training** is essential in the nursing profession. It ensures that caregivers keep up to date with the latest innovations, master new tools and technologies, improve their people and interpersonal skills, and grow in their careers. By investing in continuing education, caregivers not only improve the quality of care they provide, but also enhance their own job satisfaction, while ensuring a safer, more humane care environment for patients.

○ Participate in training sessions on new technologies

Taking part in training courses on new technologies has become a must for healthcare professionals, and especially for nursing assistants. Not only do these courses provide the skills needed to handle modern technological tools, they are also an opportunity to adapt to the profound changes affecting the medical field. The integration of technology into care has considerably altered the way patients are cared for, from medical monitoring to surgical interventions. For a caregiver, training in new technologies is essential to keep pace with advances, optimize the quality of care and ensure better collaboration with the medical team.

One of the main reasons why it's crucial to take part in training courses on new technologies is the **constant evolution of medical devices** used in hospitals and care centers. Equipment such as **vital monitoring devices, intelligent infusion pumps** and **vital signs monitors are becoming** increasingly sophisticated. These devices, although indispensable for patient monitoring, require technical expertise to be used to optimum effect. Training courses enable caregivers to understand how to set up and use these devices with precision, and how to correctly interpret the information provided to detect any signs of deterioration in the patient's condition.

In particular, connected monitoring devices, which enable real-time monitoring of patients' vital parameters, represent a major advance in care management. By sending automatic alerts in the event of anomalies, these devices increase the responsiveness of care teams. However, to take full advantage of these tools, the caregiver must be able to **react quickly** to these alerts, **check** the systems in the event of malfunction, and transmit the relevant information to the medical team. Training in these new technologies is therefore crucial to ensure that these devices are used safely and effectively.

Another area in which technology is transforming medical practice is **surgical robotics**, with systems such as the **Da Vinci robot**. Although it is the surgeon who directly controls the robot during the operation, nursing assistants play a key role in equipment preparation, patient positioning and intraoperative monitoring. Training in robotic technologies enables them to understand the specifics of these operations, and to assist the surgical team with greater precision and efficiency. By learning how to configure robotic arms, ensure their correct positioning and manage instruments during the operation, the caregiver actively contributes to the success of these complex procedures.

In addition to the technologies used in the operating theatre or intensive care unit, **telemedicine** represents another major transformation in the medical landscape. With the accelerating adoption of remote consultations, caregivers also need to be trained in the use of telemedicine platforms and digital tools that facilitate communication between patients and doctors. Participating in telemedicine training courses enables caregivers to master these tools, help patients connect to these platforms, guide them in managing their digital medical records, and ensure that remote consultations run smoothly. In addition, by being trained in these tools, caregivers can play a **pivotal** role between face-to-face and online consultations, facilitating continuity of care.

Beyond the technical aspects, these training courses on new technologies also enable caregivers to better understand the **impact of data** in the healthcare field. With the rise of electronic medical records, remote monitoring and connected devices, the management and protection of patient data have become crucial issues. Training in these technologies often includes awareness of **data confidentiality** and **security** issues, a fundamental aspect to be mastered to ensure compliance with health information protection standards. By understanding the issues involved in system security and data protection, caregivers play an active role in preventing cyber-attacks or leaks of sensitive information.

Training in new technologies also offers the opportunity to **develop cross-disciplinary skills**, which can be beneficial to the caregiver's professional development. For example, in-depth training in medical imaging systems such as **CT**, **MRI** or **ultrasound** provides additional expertise in assisting with the performance of these examinations, while offering the possibility of specializing in certain services. Similarly, mastery of complex monitoring devices or surgical robotics tools can open up prospects for advancement into positions of greater responsibility, such as technical assistant in operating theatres or intensive care units.

By taking part in these training courses, caregivers also gain **confidence** in the use of new technologies. This reduces the apprehensions associated with adopting new tools, and facilitates the integration of these innovations into daily practice. Indeed, unfamiliarity with technologies can sometimes be a source of stress, especially in contexts where speed of execution and precision are crucial, such as the emergency room or operating theatre. Training courses provide a safe learning environment, where caregivers can practice handling devices without pressure, ask questions, and gradually familiarize themselves with new systems before using them in the field.

Finally, the importance of such training goes beyond technical improvement: it also enhances the **quality of care** provided to patients. By being trained in the latest innovations, caregivers are better equipped to understand the benefits of these technologies for the patient, whether in terms of safety, comfort or care efficiency. For example, the use of **intelligent infusion pumps** enables medication to be administered with greater precision, reducing the risk of medication errors. Similarly, advanced monitoring devices enable earlier detection of complications, improving the chances of rapid intervention in the event of a problem. By being trained in these tools, caregivers contribute directly to improving patient care, by ensuring that technologies are used optimally.

Chapter 7

Ethical issues in urology care

Respect the patient's dignity in all circumstances
　　　　◦　　Managing delicate situations during intimate care
Managing delicate situations during intimate care is a fundamental part of the nursing profession. This care, which includes gestures as varied as intimate grooming, catheter insertion or the monitoring of medical devices such as catheters, touches directly on the modesty, intimacy and sometimes the dignity of patients. Because of their deeply personal nature, these procedures can be a source of embarrassment or discomfort for patients and caregivers alike. It is therefore essential to approach such care with **great sensitivity**, **irreproachable professionalism**, and **constant respect** for patients' values and emotions.

The first key to managing these situations is **communication**, which must be clear, empathetic and adapted to each patient. Before performing any intimate care, it's crucial to explain to the patient what we're going to do, why it's necessary, and how it's going to be carried out. Good communication can **defuse** some of the anxiety or discomfort felt by the patient. It's important to use simple, reassuring terms, and always ensure that the patient has understood and given his or her consent. For example, before performing an intimate cleansing or inserting a urinary catheter, the caregiver can explain the purpose of the procedure, stressing that it is part of the care required to ensure the patient's health and comfort. By anticipating the patient's questions or concerns, the caregiver creates a climate of trust.

Respect for modesty is a priority in all intimate care. Even if the patient's body is often very exposed during such care, it is essential to always preserve as much privacy as possible. This may involve simple but essential gestures, such as covering the patient with a towel or sheet, revealing only the part of the body that requires treatment. For example, during an intimate cleansing, one part of the body can be covered while the other is being washed, making the patient feel less vulnerable. This attention to physical intimacy is particularly important for patients who may already feel weakened by their illness or hospitalization.

144

It is also essential to **respect the** patient's **rhythm** and preferences. Some patients may be particularly uncomfortable with certain types of intimate care, whether for cultural, religious or personal reasons. Caregivers must be sensitive to these concerns, and always respect the patient's wishes wherever possible. For example, a patient may prefer to be cared for by a person of the same sex, or express the wish to perform some of his or her own intimate hygiene. In such cases, it's important to support the patient without forcing them to accept care they don't feel comfortable with, while explaining the possible alternatives. This flexible approach helps reduce the patient's **emotional discomfort**.

Intimate care also requires **genuine empathy**. For many patients, the loss of autonomy and the need for intimate care can be experienced as an affront to their dignity. They may feel embarrassed, vulnerable, even ashamed. The caregiver must be able to recognize these emotions and **accompany** them **with sensitivity**, without ever trivializing the situation. It may be helpful to remind the patient that these gestures are an integral part of their recovery or comfort, and that there is no shame in receiving this care. A calm, caring and respectful attitude is essential to help the patient feel supported.

Active listening also plays a central role in managing intimate care. Sometimes, patients may express fears or misgivings about their bodies or the way they perceive care. It's important to take the time to listen to their concerns and respond with care. For example, if a patient expresses pain or discomfort during care, the caregiver must be responsive by immediately adjusting his or her approach, or by seeking the advice of a nurse or doctor. This attention to the patient's voice reinforces their sense of control and respect in a situation where they may feel powerless.

The **professional attitude** is paramount during intimate care. Even though the situation may be delicate, it's important for the caregiver to maintain a neutral, benevolent approach, focused on the task in hand. This means never showing discomfort or embarrassment, even if the patient expresses embarrassment or discomfort. By maintaining a respectful, patient-focused demeanor, the caregiver helps to normalize the situation, which can help to dispel negative feelings associated with intimate care.

In some cases, it may be necessary to manage more intense **emotional reactions** on the part of patients, particularly when intimate care revives past traumas or painful experiences. If a patient seems particularly upset or anxious during such care, the caregiver must be able to adapt by taking more time to reassure, and by respecting the limits set by the patient. In such cases, it may also be advisable to call on a psychologist or a member of the medical team specializing in psychological support to offer additional support.

Respect for cultural and religious practices is also fundamental to intimate care. In some cultures, there are strict rules governing modesty or the management of the body, and it is essential that the caregiver is aware of these specificities and respects them. For example, in some religious traditions, it may be preferable for a patient to be cared for by a health professional of the same sex, or for certain treatments to be carried out under specific conditions of confidentiality. The caregiver must therefore be aware of cultural practices and ensure that they are respected as far as possible, in dialogue with the patient and his or her family.

Finally, intimate care management includes particular attention to **preserving the patient's dignity**. It's not simply a question of providing physical care, but of ensuring that every gesture is carried out with the utmost respect for the individual. This may involve simple gestures, such as asking permission before touching a part of the body, or reassuring words that show the patient we understand the sensitivity of the situation. The aim is for the patient to feel humanely treated, whatever the care provided.

◦ Ensuring the confidentiality of medical data

Ensuring the **confidentiality of medical data** is a fundamental responsibility for all healthcare professionals, and caregivers play an essential role in this. Whether it concerns a patient's state of health, their medical history or the care they receive, this data is some of the most sensitive information available. It directly affects patients' privacy and is protected by strict laws, such as the **General Data Protection Regulation (GDPR)** in Europe. Guaranteeing the confidentiality of medical data is not just a legal obligation, but also a question of ethics and respect for patients' rights. Caregivers must implement a series of rigorous practices to protect this information at every stage of its handling, from collection to archiving.

The **first step** in ensuring the confidentiality of medical data is to understand the importance of **protecting personal information**. Caregivers, who are often on the front line of patient relations, have access to a great deal of sensitive information: current treatments, test results, medical history. It is crucial to always bear in mind that this data belongs to the patient, and should only be shared within a strictly necessary and legitimate framework, i.e. only with members of the healthcare team directly involved in the patient's care. This includes doctors, nurses and other healthcare professionals involved in diagnosis and care.

Information sharing within the medical team must be discreet and secure. This means that any discussion of a patient's condition should take place in a **private space**, away from prying ears. For example, talking about a patient's care in a corridor or common room where others can hear is unacceptable. Caregivers must ensure that information is exchanged in appropriate places, such as meeting rooms or doctors' offices, to avoid any uncontrolled leakage of information.

Medical records management is another key step in ensuring data confidentiality. Increasingly, healthcare establishments are moving towards **digitizing medical records**, making data protection even more crucial, as information is now stored in electronic form. Caregivers, while not always responsible for direct access to these records, need to know how to consult or manipulate this information securely. This includes using strong passwords to access computer systems, logging off computers after use, and using medical records management software that complies with the strictest security standards.

In cases where **paper medical data** is still used, it is essential to ensure that these documents are **properly archived**. Paper files should be stored in locked cabinets, accessible only to authorized personnel. It's also important never to leave medical documents lying around in accessible areas, such as a waiting room or shared office. By handling these documents with care, caregivers help to preserve patient confidentiality.

One of today's challenges in protecting medical data lies in the use of **new technologies**. With the emergence of telemedicine, connected devices and healthcare applications, medical data is increasingly circulating in digital environments. Caregivers need to familiarize themselves with these tools and ensure that they are used in a secure manner. For example, when a patient uses an app to track his or her treatment or health parameters, it is essential that caregivers ensure that these apps comply with data protection standards. In addition, when remote consultations are carried out, the environment must be controlled to ensure that information exchanged cannot be intercepted by unauthorized third parties.

It is also crucial to respect the principles of **non-disclosure**. As a healthcare professional, it can be tempting to share details of particular clinical cases with other colleagues or friends, outside the medical setting. However, even if this is done without malicious intent, it constitutes a breach of confidentiality. It is essential to always remember that patient confidentiality is sacred, and that no information, no matter how innocuous it may seem, should be shared outside the strictly professional and medical context.

Patient consent is another fundamental element in ensuring the confidentiality of patient data. Before sharing medical information with a third party, such as a family member or another healthcare professional not directly involved in care, it is imperative to ensure that the patient has given informed consent. This consent must be obtained in a clear and documented manner, and must be respected in all circumstances. For example, a patient may choose not to share certain information with his or her family, even when hospitalized. The caregiver must respect this decision and ensure that the patient's wishes are followed to the letter.

Ongoing training plays a key role in protecting medical data. Laws and technologies are evolving rapidly, and it's crucial that caregivers are regularly trained in new security practices and regulations. Training sessions on data management, cybersecurity and information confidentiality need to be organized in healthcare establishments, so that every member of staff, including orderlies, is up to date with best practice. This training also raises awareness of the importance of these issues, which are sometimes relegated to the background in the stress of everyday life.

Finally, it is important to **report any incidents** or breaches of confidentiality. If a caregiver becomes aware that an error has been made - such as the inadvertent disclosure of medical information to an unauthorized person, or the loss of sensitive documents - he or she should immediately inform his or her supervisor or the facility's data management team. The error must be corrected as quickly as possible to minimize potential damage and prevent recurrence.

- ○ Adapting one's behavior to the patient's beliefs and values

Adapting one's behavior to the patient's beliefs and values is a fundamental requirement in the healthcare relationship. Every patient arrives with his or her own personal baggage, shaped by culture, religious beliefs, moral values and life experience. These elements influence not only their perception of illness and care, but also their expectations of the nursing staff. For a caregiver, knowing how to take these aspects into account is essential for offering respectful, individualized and truly patient-centered care. This approach not only enhances the quality of care, but also helps to establish a relationship of trust, by showing the patient that he or she is considered in his or her entirety, with his or her specificities and choices.

One of the first steps in adapting one's behavior is to **understand the patient's beliefs and values**. Each individual has his or her own perception of health, illness, pain or death, depending on his or her cultural and religious background. For example, some cultures value patient autonomy and advocate individual decisions, while in others, the family plays a central role in decision-making. Certain religions can influence the way a patient approaches pain or medical treatment. For example, in some traditions, suffering may be seen as a spiritual ordeal to be endured, which may lead the patient to refuse certain pain treatments. It is essential for the caregiver to **be aware of** these specificities, to listen carefully to the expectations and beliefs expressed by the patient, and to respect them as far as possible.

Respect for religious practices is an essential dimension of this adaptation. Some religions impose specific rules concerning diet, body care or the gender of the caregiver. For example, a Muslim patient may have preferences concerning the way in which care is provided, particularly with regard to modesty and intimate hygiene. In this case, the caregiver should respect the patient's request to receive care from a person of the same gender if possible. Similarly, some Jewish patients may have dietary restrictions, especially on certain religious holidays such as the Sabbath or Yom Kippur. In such cases, it is the caregiver's duty to ensure that these requests are taken into account in the meals served at the hospital, in collaboration with the nutrition team.

Another important dimension is **respect for rituals and spiritual practices**. Some patients may need to pray at specific times of the day, receive a visit from a religious minister, or practice certain rites during their hospital stay. It is essential to respect these practices, which often play a crucial role in the patient's emotional and spiritual well-being. The caregiver can facilitate these moments by ensuring that the patient has a quiet space in which to pray, or by informing the hospital's religious service so that a priest, imam, rabbi or other spiritual representative can intervene if the patient so wishes. **Listening to spiritual needs** in this way shows patients that their religious dimension is not only accepted, but also valued as part of their care.

In addition to religious beliefs, the patient's **personal values** must also be respected. These values can influence crucial choices, such as the acceptance or refusal of certain treatments. For example, some patients may refuse blood transfusions for religious reasons, like Jehovah's Witnesses. Others may choose alternative or natural treatments to complement traditional medicine, depending on their vision of the body and healing. Although often faced with choices that differ from medical recommendations, the caregiver must adopt a **non-judgmental attitude**, respecting the patient's autonomy and right to decide. By facilitating communication between the patient, his or her family and the medical team, the caregiver can help find a compromise that respects the patient's values while guaranteeing his or her safety.

Active listening is another valuable tool for adapting behavior. Every patient is unique, and although generalities may apply to certain cultures or beliefs, it's important not to make assumptions. The caregiver must take the time to talk with the patient to understand his or her specific expectations. Sometimes, patients may be reluctant to express their needs, for fear of being disturbed or misunderstood. The caregiver, by creating a climate of trust and dialogue, enables the patient to feel comfortable talking about his or her beliefs or values, and thus ensures that these aspects are taken into account in his or her care.

Language and communication also play a central role in behavioral adaptation. For some patients, language barriers can make it difficult to understand medical care or procedures. In such cases, it is essential for the caregiver to ensure that translation tools are available, whether an interpreter or translated documents. Furthermore, some cultures attach great importance to the way patients are addressed. In some Asian cultures, for example, respect for elders is paramount, and a respectful tone of voice and courteous gestures are essential to establishing a good care relationship. Adapting one's language to the patient's cultural sensitivity helps to better understand him or her and reduce misunderstandings.

Palliative or end-of-life care is a particularly delicate context in which patients' beliefs and values take on crucial importance. At such times, **spirituality** and religious beliefs often play a central role for patients and their families. Some patients may wish to follow particular rites or spiritual practices before they die. The caregiver must be ready to support these requests, whether they involve the presence of a chaplain, a special prayer or certain funeral rituals. Respecting these wishes is fundamental to enabling the patient to live through this stage with dignity and serenity, in accordance with his or her values.

In addition to religious or spiritual care, **adapting day-to-day care** is also essential. For example, some patients may hold beliefs about the integrity of the body, and be reluctant to undergo certain procedures, such as the insertion of a urinary catheter or the use of psychotropic drugs. In such cases, it is important to take the time to explain to the patient why these procedures are necessary, while respecting his or her right to refuse certain care. The caregiver's role is to inform without imposing, and to enable the patient to make informed decisions, while respecting his or her personal beliefs and values.

Finally, adapting one's behavior also involves **self-reflection**. Caregivers must be aware of their own beliefs, values and prejudices, and take care not to project them onto patients. It can sometimes be difficult to understand or accept certain life or health choices that differ from one's own. However, the duty of

152

the caregiver is to adopt a professional, respectful and open attitude. This ability to detach oneself from one's own convictions in order to better understand those of others is a sign of professional maturity and empathy.

Ethical dilemmas specific to urology
    ◦   Informed consent for invasive procedures

Informed consent is a fundamental principle in medicine, and is particularly important when it comes to **invasive procedures**. These procedures, which may include surgery, punctures, biopsies or the insertion of medical devices such as catheters or probes, involve a degree of risk and often affect the patient's physical integrity. Before any invasive procedure is carried out, it is essential that the patient is fully informed of what is involved, and gives informed consent. This process is not just a legal formality: it is based on **trusting dialogue**, **clear information** and full respect for the patient's right to actively participate in his or her own care.

Informed consent is based first and foremost on the idea that patients have the right to control their own bodies and make decisions about their health. It's not simply a matter of informing the patient that a procedure is going to take place, but of explaining in detail what is involved, so that he or she can make a well-considered, conscious decision. This includes not only the **potential benefits of** the procedure, but also the **risks**, possible **alternatives**, as well as the **consequences** of not carrying it out. For example, before undergoing urological surgery such as prostatectomy, it is imperative that the patient understands not only the purpose of the operation, but also the possible complications, such as impaired continence or erectile function.

The caregiver's role in this process is often indirect, but nonetheless crucial. Although consent is usually obtained by the doctor, the caregiver plays an important role in **accompanying** the patient and **answering** any **questions** he or she may have before or after the doctor's explanation. Patients may sometimes hesitate to ask their doctor questions, but feel more at ease with the caregiver. The caregiver can then act as an intermediary, clarifying certain points or encouraging the patient to express his or her concerns. This is a time of great vulnerability for the patient, and the caregiver, by listening and supporting the patient, helps to create an environment where the patient feels safe to ask for more information if he or she does not understand certain aspects of the procedure.

The **information provided** to obtain informed consent must be **clear**, **accessible** and, above all, adapted to the patient's level of understanding. Some medical terms or technical concepts may be difficult for patients to understand, and it is the caregiver's responsibility to ensure that each piece of information is explained in an understandable way. This may involve simplifying explanations or using analogies that enable the patient to better visualize what is going to happen. For example, rather than using the term "ablation" when referring to a surgical procedure, the caregiver may simply explain that it involves removing part of an organ or tumor. The caregiver can play a key role in this process, being alert to any signs of confusion or misunderstanding on the part of the patient.

Informed consent must also be **voluntary**. The aim is not to pressure the patient into accepting a treatment or procedure, but to give him or her all the information needed to make a free and informed decision. It is essential to respect the patient's choice, even if it runs counter to medical recommendations. The patient may, for example, refuse to undergo surgery, even if it is deemed necessary by the doctor. In such situations, it is crucial that the caregiver remains judgmental-non, and continues to support the patient throughout the care process. Refusal of consent is a fundamental right, and patients must be informed of the possible consequences of their choice, without pressure or coercion.

An essential aspect of informed consent is that it is **not set in stone**. The patient has the right to change his or her mind at any time. They may initially agree to a procedure, but later wish to refuse it. In this case, it is important that the care team, including the caregiver, remains attentive and respects this decision. For example, a patient who has consented to the insertion of a urinary catheter may, at the last moment, express reluctance. It is the caregiver's responsibility to listen to these doubts, answer their questions and, if necessary, delay or cancel the procedure, until the patient has again given informed consent.

It's also important to note that certain situations can complicate obtaining informed consent, particularly when the patient is **vulnerable** or unable to understand the information provided. This may include elderly patients suffering from dementia, people with cognitive disorders or unconscious patients. In these cases, consent must be obtained from a **legal guardian** or family members, according to the rules in force. The caregiver must then ensure that the designated person receives the same detailed information and is able to make a decision in the patient's best interests.

Time is also of the essence in obtaining informed consent. Patients must have sufficient time to reflect on their decision, without feeling pressured to respond immediately. It is important that caregivers, and in particular orderlies, allow the patient to ask questions at different times, to consult relatives or to take time to reflect before signing a consent document. The caregiver's support can be invaluable here, to ensure that the patient has had the opportunity to assimilate the information.

Finally, informed consent is more than just a **signed document**. Although signing a form is often a necessary step, informed consent is first and foremost an **ongoing process of** communication and clarification. The signed document is a legal formality, but it must be preceded by in-depth discussion and followed by regular checks to ensure that the patient has fully understood and continues to consent to the care provided.

○ End-of-life and palliative care issues

The **issues surrounding end-of-life and palliative care** are among the most complex and delicate in the medical field. These issues touch directly on human dignity, individual choice and support for terminally ill patients and their families. Palliative care, which aims to provide pain relief and comfort, focuses on improving quality of life rather than curing. It raises medical, ethical and psychological challenges that must be approached with sensitivity and empathy. The caregiver, in the front line of this accompaniment, plays a crucial role in providing physical and emotional support to the patient and his or her loved ones, while managing the practical aspects of this particular care.

One of the **first issues** surrounding the end-of-life phase is the question of **psychological and emotional support** for patients. In the terminal phase, patients are often confronted with feelings of fear, anxiety, sadness or uncertainty in the face of imminent death. The role of caregivers is to provide constant **emotional support**, creating an environment where the patient feels listened to, respected and understood. This requires active listening, but also a great ability to adapt to the specific needs of each patient. Some patients may seek to discuss death openly, express their anxieties or evoke regrets or hopes, while others prefer to avoid these subjects and concentrate on the practical aspects of everyday life.

In these moments, the caregiver must be able to **respect the** patient's **rhythm** and adapt to his or her emotional needs, without imposing a discourse or vision. The caregiver must also be attentive to non-verbal suffering, as some patients, particularly those who are debilitated or losing communication, may express their pain or anguish through gestures, looks or behavior. Being present, even in silence, can offer invaluable support.

Another central issue is **pain management** in palliative care. At the end of life, physical pain can become intense and requires specialized management. Painkillers, such as morphine or other opioids, are often needed to alleviate this pain, but this sometimes raises ethical questions concerning the doses administered, particularly when these drugs can alter the patient's state of consciousness or indirectly shorten his or her life. The caregiver's role here is to **monitor** pain **symptoms**, promptly report any signs of deterioration, and actively participate in the administration of comfort care, such as repositioning the patient, applying relaxation techniques or hydration. The aim is to offer **optimal quality of life**, despite the severity of the situation.

At the same time, it's essential to ensure **transparent, caring communication** with the family. The end of life is a particularly trying time for loved ones, who are often confronted with ambivalent feelings: sadness at the impending loss, the pain of seeing a loved one suffer, but also, sometimes, the relief of knowing that this suffering will come to an end. The caregiver plays a key role in listening to families' concerns, explaining ongoing care and helping them to better understand the process. Some family members may have unrealistic expectations about how the situation will evolve, or hope for improbable improvements. The caregiver, while showing empathy, must help manage these expectations, while respecting their need for hope and support.

Palliative care also raises complex **ethical issues**, particularly with regard to patient autonomy and end-of-life decisions. Many patients express **advance directives**, i.e. wishes concerning the care they do or do not wish to receive as they approach death. These directives can include decisions such as refusing to be overly aggressive, not wanting to be resuscitated in the event of cardiac arrest, or requesting deep and continuous sedation to relieve pain. Respecting these wishes is fundamental, but they can sometimes conflict with the values of loved ones or with medical considerations. Although not a decision-maker in such cases, the caregiver must **ensure that the patient's wishes are respected**, by ensuring that these decisions are respected by the care team and the family.

The **role of spirituality** is also a key dimension of end-of-life care. For many patients, the question of death is deeply linked to their religious or spiritual beliefs. Some may wish to be visited by a chaplain or religious representative, participate in spiritual rites or prayers, while others may need a space to meditate or reflect. The caregiver must ensure that these needs are respected, by facilitating access to spiritual guidance and creating an environment conducive to spirituality, whether through simple gestures such as lighting a candle, offering a prayer book or allowing a loved one to visit for a blessing.

Palliative care also raises the question of patient **autonomy and dignity**. As the disease progresses, patients can lose their autonomy, which can be a source of frustration and moral suffering. The caregiver must therefore find ways of **preserving the** patient's **dignity** by respecting his or her autonomy as far as possible, even in the small things of everyday life: letting the patient choose when to wash up, deciding how he or she wants to be seated, or encouraging him or her to carry out gestures that he or she can still do themselves, even if they are limited. Maintaining these moments of control is crucial to the patient's esteem-self and sense of humanity.

Finally, palliative care support does not end with the patient's death. The **mourning** period is an essential stage, for families and caregivers alike. After the death, the caregiver must be there to support the loved ones, listening to them, answering their questions and helping them through the first moments of grief. It may also be necessary to take a moment for themselves, as accompanying a patient to his or her death is an emotionally intense experience, which can leave a deep imprint on caregivers. It is important for caregivers to benefit from **psychological support** or moments of exchange with their colleagues to share their emotions and avoid burnout.

- ◦ Handling requests from patients who disagree with medical practices

Dealing with requests from patients who disagree with medical practices is a delicate task, requiring a great deal of listening, understanding and diplomacy on the part of caregivers, especially orderlies. Because of their personal, religious or cultural beliefs, or their past experiences, patients may sometimes refuse or contest certain treatments proposed by the medical team. Such disagreement may concern specific medical procedures, drug treatments, or even interventions deemed necessary by doctors, such as blood transfusions or surgery. When faced with such situations, it is essential to respect the patient's choices, while seeking to find common ground that safeguards his or her health and safety.

The **first step** in managing these disagreements is to adopt an **attitude of active listening**. When a patient expresses refusal to undergo a treatment or procedure, it is crucial not to react with judgment or imposition. The caregiver must first try to understand the reasons for this refusal by letting the patient express himself. Patients may have fears or misunderstandings about the proposed procedure, or cultural or religious beliefs that dictate their choices. By taking the time to listen without interrupting, the caregiver shows the patient that his or her opinion is being taken into account, which often helps to **defuse a tense situation**.

A **clear and sympathetic explanation** of why treatment is recommended can then be given. One of the main challenges when patients refuse certain care is that they don't always understand the necessity or consequences of their decision. For example, a patient may refuse a minor surgical procedure for fear of complications, without understanding that it could prevent more serious problems in the long term. The caregiver, like the doctor, has a pedagogical role to play in explaining in a simple and accessible way why the proposed treatment is important. In this process, it is essential to avoid overly complex technical terms and to adapt the discourse to the patient's level of understanding, while respecting his or her need for clarification.

It is also crucial to **respect patient autonomy**. Every individual has the right to control his or her own body and to make decisions concerning his or her health, even if these go against medical recommendations. This respect for autonomy is enshrined in the ethical principles of modern medicine, and also applies to situations where the patient makes choices that are not deemed medically optimal. The caregiver must therefore respect these decisions without passing judgment, ensuring that the patient is fully informed of the risks involved in refusing treatment. For example, a cancer patient may refuse chemotherapy because of its side effects, preferring to opt for alternative treatments. In this situation, it is the caregiver's duty to support the patient in his or her choices, while ensuring that the patient is fully aware of the consequences of refusing treatment.

In some situations, disagreement may stem from specific **religious beliefs**, such as the refusal of blood transfusions by Jehovah's Witnesses. These beliefs, although they may seem incompatible with medical practice, must be respected. The caregiver, in collaboration with the medical team, can then explore **alternatives to** meet the patient's needs while respecting his or her convictions. For example, in the case of a patient refusing a transfusion, it may be possible to discuss with the doctor the options of autologous blood recovery or other solutions that avoid the need for a transfusion. The caregiver's role here is to **facilitate dialogue** between the patient and the healthcare team, ensuring that the patient feels heard and respected.

Family involvement is often a key element in managing disagreements. Some patients, particularly those at the end of life or suffering from chronic illnesses, can be influenced by the opinions of their loved ones. Sometimes, the family itself may disagree with medical recommendations and seek to influence the patient's decisions. In such cases, the caregiver must be **diplomatic**, respecting family dynamics while ensuring that the patient's choices are respected. It is essential to **clarify** with the patient what his or her wishes **are**, and to ensure that he or she is not under pressure from relatives. If tensions arise, the caregiver can encourage a discussion with the medical team to promote open dialogue between the patient, family and caregivers.

When disagreement persists, it's important to know **when to escalate the situation**. If a patient refuses treatment that could endanger his or her life or seriously compromise his or her health, it is essential that the caregiver alerts the doctor or nurse in charge so that they can take the necessary action. The patient must be reassessed and formally informed by the doctor of the risks involved. In certain situations, **legal action** may be taken if the patient is deemed incapable of making informed decisions, or is unknowingly endangering his or her own safety. However, such measures are rare and must always respect the patient's autonomy and dignity.

Managing the demands of patients who disagree with medical practices also raises **ethical issues**. Caregivers are often torn between their duty to care and their obligation to respect patients' choices. This tension can be difficult to live with, as it confronts the caregiver with moral dilemmas. In such situations, it is useful for caregivers to be able to **discuss** these dilemmas **with their colleagues** at team meetings, or to seek the advice of the establishment's ethics committee, if possible. It is important for caregivers to be supported in managing these complex situations, and to have the resources they need to navigate these grey areas.

Finally, we must never lose sight of the importance of **caring**. Patients who refuse certain types of care do not do so out of defiance, but often out of fear, incomprehension or because of values they hold dear. By maintaining an open, non-judgmental and respectful attitude, the caregiver helps to **preserve the relationship of trust** with the patient, even in situations of disagreement. This bond of trust is crucial if the caregiver is to continue to accompany the patient on his or her care journey, even if the patient chooses a different path to that advocated by medicine.

The ethics of new technologies in urology

  ◦   The impact of robots and artificial intelligence on the caregiver-patient relationship

The **impact of robots and artificial intelligence (AI) on the caregiver-patient relationship** is a topic of great importance as these technologies become increasingly integrated into the medical field. While these technological advances offer impressive possibilities for improving the precision of care, reducing human error and optimizing task management, they also raise crucial questions about the human aspect of care. The caregiver-patient relationship, traditionally based on trust, empathy and communication, can be profoundly altered by the introduction of automated and intelligent technologies. Caregivers need to find a new balance between the use of these tools and the maintenance of the human bond that is essential to quality care.

One of the **major advantages** of robots and artificial intelligence is their ability to **improve the efficiency** and **precision** of care. In fields such as surgery, the use of robots such as the Da Vinci robot enables surgeons to perform operations with millimetric precision, reducing the risk of complications. AIs, meanwhile, play a crucial role in diagnosis, medical image analysis, and even predicting patient health trajectories by analyzing large quantities of data. This frees up time for caregivers, who can devote more time to supporting patients, listening to their needs and managing their overall well-being. However, it is important to ensure that these technologies do not **detract from the human presence** essential to a quality care relationship.

The **risk of a dehumanization of** care is often evoked with the massive introduction of robotic technologies and AI. Patients, especially those in fragile situations, need to feel a human presence, to know that they are being listened to and understood by a caregiver capable of responding to their emotional, and not just medical, needs. The danger of relying excessively on robots or AI would be to create a distance between patient and caregiver, where interactions become more mechanical and impersonal. For example, the use of AI to carry out diagnoses or consultations online, while convenient and fast, can leave patients in a situation where they feel disconnected from a real human interlocutor, which can lead to **feelings of isolation** or a loss of trust in the healthcare system.

The **relationship of trust** between patient and caregiver relies heavily on communication and empathy, two aspects that technology cannot replace. Robots and AI are very good at analyzing data, detecting anomalies or providing automated treatments, but they cannot, to date, recreate the **humanity** that lies at the heart of the caregiver-patient relationship. Patients often seek to understand their state of health not only through technical explanations, but also through personal exchanges, advice tailored to their situation, and the moral support that only a human being can offer. Caregivers must therefore ensure that the use of robotic or intelligent technologies does not encroach on these crucial moments of interaction, where listening and reassurance are essential.

It's also important to point out that the introduction of robots and AI into the medical field can sometimes create **apprehension** in some patients. Not everyone is comfortable with the idea of receiving care from a machine or entrusting part of their treatment to an algorithm. It can be perceived as a loss of control or a dehumanization of the care process. In this context, the role of caregivers is all the more important: they need to **reassure patients**, explain the benefits of the technologies used, and stay by their side to answer their questions and concerns. It's essential that patients understand that these technologies are there to **assist** caregivers, not replace them.

However, it is undeniable that robots and artificial intelligence bring many **benefits** which, used correctly, can enrich the caregiver-patient relationship. For example, in the field of **telemedicine**, AI makes it possible to rapidly analyze symptoms remotely, facilitating access to care for patients who live in remote areas or have difficulty travelling. This can enable caregivers to focus more on more complex aspects of care, while still offering a human presence when needed. What's more, robots can be used to perform repetitive or cumbersome tasks, such as transporting patients or managing certain procedures, freeing up caregivers for activities that require more human contact.

One of the most striking examples of this complementarity is the use of **assistance robots** in long-term care units or retirement homes. These robots can help caregivers by performing tasks such as lifting patients, dispensing medication, or even interacting with patients to stimulate them cognitively. However, these robots do not replace the emotional and affective bond that a caregiver can offer. They should be seen as **supportive tools**, enabling caregivers to focus on deeper interactions with patients, rather than being consumed by technical or logistical tasks.

It's also important to emphasize that robots and artificial intelligence can enhance the **personalization of care**, a crucial aspect of the caregiver-patient relationship. By analyzing healthcare data on a large scale, AIs can propose treatments tailored to each patient's specific needs, taking into account their medical history, preferences and lifestyle. Caregivers can thus better tailor care to each patient, offering a more individualized approach. However, this algorithm-based personalization must always be accompanied by the **clinical judgment** of the caregiver, who remains indispensable for interpreting AI recommendations in the light of the patient's human and emotional context.

○ The ethics of genetic sequencing and sensitive data
The **ethics of genetic sequencing** and the management of the resulting **sensitive data** are fundamental issues in modern medicine. Advances in DNA sequencing technologies have made it possible to map the human genome with unprecedented precision, opening up extraordinary prospects for the prevention, diagnosis and treatment of disease. However, this genetic revolution is accompanied by numerous ethical questions, notably concerning confidentiality, respect for privacy, the use of genetic

data, and the risks of discrimination. These issues raise complex questions about how this sensitive information should be managed, shared and protected.

Genetic sequencing involves analyzing an individual's genes to identify mutations or genetic variations that may predispose to certain diseases or influence response to treatment. This makes it possible to anticipate the risk of hereditary diseases such as certain cancers, to diagnose rare genetic disorders or to adapt treatments to the patient's genetic particularities, in what is known as **personalized medicine**. While these advances represent a major step forward for healthcare, they also raise crucial questions about the use of this genetic information.

One of the first ethical issues raised by genetic sequencing is that of **data confidentiality**. Genetic sequencing produces extremely sensitive data, revealing profound information about an individual's biological identity, as well as that of those close to him or her. Unlike simple medical test results, genetic data can reveal predispositions to diseases that may never manifest themselves, but which also concern family members who share the same genetic heritage. **Particular care** must therefore be taken when handling this information, to ensure that it is not used for purposes that could be harmful to the individual.

The **risk of discrimination** is one of the major concerns in the use of genetic data. For example, if a person is identified as carrying a gene that increases their risk of developing a serious disease, such as Alzheimer's or cancer, they could be discriminated against in the context of health insurance or employment, if this information is disclosed or used for non-medical purposes. Although legislation exists in many countries to protect individuals against genetic discrimination (such as the **Genetic Information Nondiscrimination Act** in the USA), there remains a risk that such data could be misused or disclosed without the patient's consent.

Informed consent is therefore at the heart of the ethical issues surrounding genetic sequencing. It is essential that every individual who agrees to have his or her genome sequenced clearly understands what is involved, not only in terms of immediate medical results, but also the long-term consequences. Consent must include explanations of how the data will be stored, who will have access to it, and for what purposes it might be used in the future, particularly in medical research. However, informed consent in this field is often complex, as it is difficult for patients to understand all the potential implications of genetic information, which may have consequences for their personal, family and professional lives.

Another important ethical issue is the **sharing of genetic data** for research purposes. Genetic sequencing generates a mass of data which, when combined on a large scale, can offer considerable opportunities for scientific discovery. For example, by analyzing the genetic data of millions of people, researchers can better understand the genetic basis of complex diseases and develop more effective treatments. However, this raises the question of the **privacy of** the individuals whose data is used. Even if this information is anonymized, there is still a risk that individuals can be re-identified from their genetic profile, especially if these data are cross-referenced with other databases.

The **right not to know** is another ethical issue raised by genetic sequencing. Some people may not want to know about their predisposition to serious or incurable diseases. For example, a person might not want to know that he or she carries a gene responsible for Huntington's disease, an incurable neurodegenerative disorder. Respecting this choice is fundamental, but it may conflict with the medical duty to inform patients of potential risks to their health or that of their family. Healthcare professionals must therefore navigate this grey area with care, ensuring that patients are fully informed of their right to choose not to be informed of certain results.

There is also the question of the **transmission of genetic information** within the family. Genetic sequencing may reveal risks for members of the patient's family, who may not be aware of these predispositions. This raises an ethical question: how far does the duty to reveal this information to relatives extend? On the one hand, it may be ethically justifiable to inform a family member of a genetic risk, so that he or she can take preventive measures. On the other hand, it could be perceived as an invasion of privacy, especially if that person does not wish to be informed. It is essential to strike a **balance** between respect for patient confidentiality and the health interests of relatives.

Finally, the ethics of genetic sequencing raise profound questions about **equal access** to these technologies. Genetic sequencing and personalized medicine offer revolutionary prospects for healthcare, but these advances are costly and not always accessible to all. This can create inequalities between those who can afford access to these technologies and those who cannot. It is therefore essential that governments and healthcare institutions work to ensure that these advances benefit the whole population, not just those who can afford them.

Chapter 8

Rare and complex pathologies in urology

Rare urological diseases: a challenge for caregivers

◦ Caring for patients with rare diseases

Caring for **patients suffering from rare diseases** represents a complex challenge for caregivers, on both medical and human levels. In the European Union, a rare disease is defined as a condition affecting less than one person in 2,000. These pathologies are often poorly understood, difficult to diagnose and treat, and require specific care adapted to the particular needs of each patient. Caring for these patients requires special attention, active listening and a multidisciplinary approach to meet the various medical, psychological and social challenges they face.

One of the first challenges in caring for patients with rare diseases is **diagnosis**. Many rare diseases are difficult to identify, due to their often atypical symptoms or slow progression. The diagnostic process can therefore be long, frustrating and sometimes exhausting for patients and their families. They may go from one doctor to another, undergoing multiple tests, without getting a clear answer. For caregivers, it is essential to accompany these patients with **empathy**, to support them during this period of uncertainty, and to work closely with specialized medical teams to speed up the diagnostic process as much as possible. The announcement of a rare disease, when it is finally made, is often experienced with a mixture of relief and anxiety in the face of the unknown. It's crucial to communicate transparently, explaining to the patient the next steps and any available treatments.

Once a diagnosis has been made, patient support must be **personalized** and tailored to the complexity of the disease. As rare diseases are by definition little studied, there are often few specific treatments, which can lead to situations of therapeutic uncertainty. In this context, a **multidisciplinary approach** is essential. Patients must be cared for by a team of specialized doctors, physiotherapists, psychologists and other healthcare professionals, depending on the manifestations of the disease. The caregiver plays a central role in this system, acting as a link between the patient and the various professionals involved, while providing basic care and ensuring the patient's comfort on a day-to-day basis.

For many rare disease patients, the care pathway can include complex, experimental or even **compassionate** treatments, i.e. administered in the absence of validated therapies. This may involve clinical trials or innovative drugs, which are often costly and difficult to access. It is essential that caregivers are well informed about available **treatment options**, that they can discuss them clearly with patients, and that they participate in the design of the care pathway in collaboration with specialist physicians. Psychological support also plays a crucial role in these situations, as the uncertainty associated with experimental treatments can generate stress and anxiety in patients and their families. Caregivers need to listen, offer answers, and refer patients to psychological support services or patient associations if necessary.

One of the special aspects of caring for patients **with** rare diseases is managing **the isolation** they may feel. Because of the rarity of their condition, patients can feel isolated, misunderstood and sometimes abandoned by the healthcare system. They are often confronted with a lack of information, or even gaps in the healthcare offer adapted to their illness. It is therefore essential to support them not only medically, but also in their **day-to-day lives**. The caregiver plays a fundamental role in providing a comforting presence, offering moral support, and fostering a care environment where patients feel recognized in their uniqueness. The caregiver can also refer patients to support groups or associations that bring together other people with the same pathology, offering an opportunity to share experiences and help each other.

Ongoing training for caregivers is also a crucial issue in the care of rare diseases. As these pathologies are often little-known and poorly documented, it is vital that caregivers, particularly nursing assistants, receive regular training to update their knowledge and adapt to changes in treatments. They must be able to adopt a proactive attitude to care management, anticipate possible complications, and work closely with specialists. The caregiver's role is not limited to performing care, but also includes **an educational accompaniment** dimension, explaining to the patient the gestures to adopt to improve his or her comfort, monitoring the effects of treatments, and ensuring that medical protocols are respected.

Another key aspect of caring for patients with rare diseases is **taking families into account**. These diseases often affect children or young adults, making family support all the more important. Families are sometimes at a loss when faced with their loved one's illness, especially when the disease is unknown or little studied. The caregiver, as a local professional, plays an **essential support** role, helping them to understand the situation, manage their stress, and organize daily life around care. Families often have to adapt to new routines, demanding treatments and home care. Caregivers can guide them through the process, teaching them technical gestures and reassuring them about their ability to support their sick loved one.

Patients suffering from rare diseases are also frequently confronted with **administrative and financial** difficulties, notably due to the high cost of treatments or medical equipment, often not reimbursed by conventional insurance schemes. Caregivers can play a mediating role by directing patients towards social services or appropriate care schemes, and helping them to put together files to access financial aid or medical assistance programs.

◦   Adapting care and protocols for specific cases

Adapting care and protocols for specific cases is an essential component of modern healthcare practice. Each patient presents a unique situation, influenced by age, general health, medical history, beliefs and specific needs. So, while standardized care protocols serve as a guide to ensure consistent and safe care, it is often necessary to adjust them to suit individual patient circumstances. This adaptability relies on the experience of caregivers, their ability to observe and understand patients' specific needs, and a multi-disciplinary approach, where each member of the medical team can contribute to refining care.

One of the first areas where care adaptation is crucial is the **management of patients with co-morbidities**. These patients often suffer from several chronic or acute illnesses simultaneously, which complicates the application of standard protocols. For example, a patient suffering from both diabetes and renal failure will have different needs to those of a patient with a single pathology. Adapting care in such cases requires careful management of drug therapy, as some drugs useful in treating one disease may aggravate another. The caregiver must be particularly vigilant for drug interactions, monitor the patient's vital signs more frequently, and work closely with other healthcare professionals to adjust treatments on a day-to-day basis. This may also involve modifying care routines, such as feeding and hydration management, to ensure that they respect the restrictions imposed by the different pathologies.

Another area where adapting care is crucial is in the **care of the elderly**, particularly those suffering from cognitive disorders such as dementia or Alzheimer's disease. These patients often exhibit unpredictable behavior, memory loss or communication difficulties, which can complicate the application of routine care. In this context, it is essential that the caregiver adapts the way he/ she interacts with the patient, using simplified communication techniques, patience and regular repetition of important information. In addition, the care environment needs to be modified to ensure the patient's safety and comfort, for example by creating more structured routines or reducing sensory stimuli that can cause confusion or anxiety. In these cases, care is not limited to technical gestures: it also encompasses an approach focused on the patient's emotional well-being and dignity.

Pediatric care, especially for **children with chronic or rare diseases**, also demands a high degree of flexibility. Children, depending on their age and development, react differently to treatments and require constant adjustments. A child suffering from cystic fibrosis, for example, will need specific care to manage respiratory secretions, diet and physical activity, as well as psychological support to help them understand their illness. The caregiver, in consultation with the medical team, will have to adapt care to the evolution of the disease, while maintaining constant dialogue with the parents, who are essential partners in the day-to-day management of the child's care. Taking psychological and family aspects into account is essential if care is to be adapted not only to the child's physical needs, but also to his or her emotional environment.

In some cases, **palliative care** also requires significant adaptation of care protocols. Terminally ill patients often have very specific needs, focused primarily on pain relief, symptom management and maintaining comfort. In these situations, standard disease treatment protocols need to be modified to focus on comfort care, not cure. Caregivers need to be alert to subtle signs of pain or discomfort, sometimes not verbalized by the patient, and adjust medication doses accordingly. In addition, it is essential to work with the patient's loved ones to understand the patient's wishes regarding the end of life, in order to adapt care while respecting each person's ethical and personal choices. Listening, being present and respecting advance directives thus become central elements in adapting care in these contexts.

Adapting care protocols is also essential for patients suffering from serious infectious diseases, such as COVID-19 or other transmissible pathologies. In these cases, care must be adapted to minimize the risk of transmission while ensuring adequate medical support. This often involves adjustments in the use of personal protective equipment (PPE), in the management of care areas, and in the way interventions are carried out. For example, a COVID-19 patient requiring respiratory assistance will need to be treated in an isolated room, with strict disinfection and waste management protocols, while benefiting from continuous monitoring of respiratory parameters. Caregivers need to be trained in specific techniques to reduce transmission while maintaining high-quality care, which requires flexibility and constant vigilance.

Another example where adapting care is crucial concerns patients with **specific cultural beliefs or practices**. Some patients, depending on their religion or culture, may refuse certain treatments, or have particular needs in terms of diet, prayer or physical contact. In such situations, the caregiver must adapt care protocols to respect the patient's beliefs, while guaranteeing his or her safety and well-being. For example, a Muslim patient may refuse treatment during the Ramadan fast, or a female patient may wish to be cared for only by female staff. The caregiver must then find solutions to respect these choices, while ensuring that the necessary care is provided in a way that respects the patient's convictions.

Finally, adapting care also involves managing **emergency situations**. Some patients, because of their fragile state of health or chronic pathologies, require specific adaptations to emergency protocols. For example, a patient with a history of cardiac or respiratory disorders may require different management in the event of cardiac arrest or respiratory distress. Adapting care in such cases requires anticipatory risk management, with rigorous preparation of possible interventions and in-depth knowledge of the specific needs of these patients in critical situations.

Complex pathologies and co-morbidities
  ◦ Managing patients with multiple chronic conditions (diabetes, hypertension, etc.)

Managing patients with multiple chronic conditions, such as diabetes, hypertension or heart failure, is a complex and demanding challenge for caregivers. These patients, often referred to as **polypathological** patients, present with several chronic illnesses simultaneously, which complicates their management.

175

Each pathology has its own requirements in terms of treatment, follow-up and prevention of complications, and a comprehensive, coordinated approach is essential to prevent the management of one disease aggravating the other. The care of these patients therefore demands special attention, vigilance and a multidisciplinary approach, in which every player in the care chain plays a crucial role in ensuring the patient's well-being.

The **complexity of interactions between pathologies** is one of the main challenges in managing these patients. For example, a diabetic patient who also suffers from high blood pressure may see his or her condition worsen if one of the diseases is not properly controlled. Diabetes, by damaging the blood vessels and kidneys, can aggravate hypertension, and conversely, poorly controlled hypertension can exacerbate diabetes-related complications, such as kidney disease. The role of caregivers is to **carefully monitor** the patient's condition, ensure rigorous follow-up of the various treatments, and report any changes in vital signs or symptoms that could indicate decompensation of one of the pathologies.

The management of polypathological patients also relies on **care coordination**. These patients are often followed by several specialists, such as a diabetologist, cardiologist, nephrologist or pulmonologist, depending on their pathologies. This multiplicity of care providers can sometimes lead to a fragmentation of care, with each specialist concentrating on his or her own specialty without necessarily having an overall view of the patient's health. It is therefore crucial that the caregiver, in particular, plays a **pivotal** role in coordinating care, ensuring that information flows smoothly between the various contributors and helping the patient to understand the sometimes contradictory or complex medical recommendations. The caregiver can also act as a relay between the various healthcare professionals, passing on key observations on the patient's condition that may require adjustments in treatment.

Medication management is another essential aspect of caring for patients with multiple chronic conditions. These patients often take a large number of medications, which exposes them to the risk of **polymedication**. Polymedication can lead to undesirable drug interactions, side effects, forgetfulness and errors in medication administration. It is therefore crucial to ensure that patients take their medication **carefully**, checking that prescribed doses are respected, and helping them to organize their daily treatment. The caregiver can play a key role in supervising medication intake, checking that the patient has understood his or her treatment regimen and helping to manage any side effects. In some cases, the caregiver can also alert the nurse or doctor to any **compliance difficulties** (such as frequent forgetfulness or confusion) that may require a reassessment of the treatment.

Another major challenge in managing polypathological patients is **preventing complications**. Every chronic disease presents risks of long-term complications, and the coexistence of several pathologies considerably increases these risks. For example, a patient suffering from diabetes and hypertension is at risk of developing cardiovascular complications, such as myocardial infarction or stroke. Preventing these complications requires **careful**, regular **monitoring of** vital parameters such as blood sugar, blood pressure and cholesterol levels. The caregiver, in collaboration with the medical team, must ensure that these parameters are rigorously monitored, by carrying out frequent checks and reporting any changes that might indicate the onset of a complication.

Lifestyle management is also a central aspect in the management of patients suffering from a number of chronic pathologies. These patients often need to adopt **lifestyle modifications**, such as a healthier diet, regular physical activity or smoking cessation, to better control their illnesses. However, these changes can be difficult to implement, especially when they concern several pathologies at the same time. For example, a diabetic patient needs to watch his or her diet to control blood sugar levels, while a hypertensive patient needs to limit salt intake to lower blood pressure. The caregiver plays a key role in the patient's **therapeutic education**, helping them to understand how these lifestyle changes can improve their health, and accompanying them as they implement these habits. It's also important to motivate patients, encourage them to persevere and help them overcome any obstacles they may encounter.

In addition to the medical aspects, the management of polypathological patients must take into account the **psychological dimension**. These patients may feel discouraged, anxious or depressed due to the constant management of their illnesses. The multiplicity of medical appointments, treatments and restrictions linked to their pathologies can generate a feeling of **mental burden** and psychological exhaustion. Because of their proximity to the patient, caregivers are often on the front line in spotting these signs of distress, and can play an important role in offering moral support, listening to the patient's concerns and, if necessary, referring them to a psychologist or psychological support service.

The care of polypathological patients also requires **constant adaptation of care** according to the evolution of illnesses and treatments. Chronic pathologies often evolve unpredictably, and it is important to regularly adjust care to meet the patient's changing needs. For example, a diabetic patient whose kidney function is deteriorating may require an adjustment in insulin treatment or changes in diet. The caregiver must remain vigilant to these changes, and be able to adapt his or her interventions accordingly, in consultation with the medical team.

Finally, **preventing hospitalization** is a key objective in the management of patients with multiple chronic pathologies. These patients are often at risk of repeated hospitalization due to the decompensation of their illnesses. One of the caregivers' priorities is therefore to **stabilize the patient's condition** as far as possible, by optimizing treatments, monitoring signs of deterioration and intervening rapidly when necessary. The caregiver, through his or her daily monitoring of the patient, plays a central role in this prevention, identifying early warning signs of complication or decompensation, and alerting health professionals before the situation requires hospitalization.

- ○ Care for frail, elderly patients

Care for frail, elderly patients requires a specific, attentive and personalized approach. With advancing age, people often become more physically and psychologically vulnerable, requiring more delicate, flexible and multidimensional care. Elderly patients may suffer from a number of chronic illnesses, diminished physical and mental capacities, or loss of autonomy. These factors contribute to making **frailty** a central element in the management of their care, where the main objective is to maintain their well-being, prevent complications and respect their dignity.

One of the key aspects of caring for frail, elderly patients is the need for a **holistic approach**. Unlike younger patients, the elderly often present with combinations of health problems. Their care cannot therefore be limited to the management of a single pathology, but must integrate all their physical, psychological and social needs. For example, an elderly patient suffering from osteoporosis, diabetes and cognitive impairment cannot be treated effectively by focusing on just one of these conditions. Every aspect of the patient's health needs to be addressed in a coherent manner. This calls for **close coordination** between the various healthcare professionals, including doctors, nurses, physiotherapists and care assistants, who play a central role in the patient's day-to-day care.

One of the main objectives in caring for elderly patients is to **preserve their autonomy** as far as possible. Even though advanced age can be accompanied by a progressive loss of certain abilities, it is essential to value and maintain remaining functions. This may involve encouraging them to carry out simple everyday tasks, such as washing, dressing or getting around, with or without assistance. Stimulating patients to be active in their own care promotes their sense of control and dignity, with beneficial effects on their morale and quality of life. The caregiver plays a crucial role in this process, **gently encouraging** the patient, adapting care to his or her abilities and providing the necessary assistance without doing everything for him or her.

Falls prevention is another crucial aspect of care for frail, elderly patients. Falls are one of the main causes of morbidity and mortality in the elderly. Due to reduced muscle strength, loss of balance and visual or cognitive impairment, elderly patients are particularly at risk. It is therefore essential to adapt the environment to make it safe: install grab bars in bathrooms, eliminate obstacles such as carpets, or ensure adequate lighting. The caregiver must also be vigilant to the patient's state of fatigue, as exhaustion can increase the risk of falling. They must adapt their care to the patient's energy level, and know how to assist them with technical aids, such as walkers or canes, to make their movements safer.

Care of elderly patients must also take into account the **cognitive disorders** common in this population, such as dementia or Alzheimer's disease. These disorders affect memory, judgment and the ability to communicate, which can make care management more complex. It is essential to adapt the way we interact with these patients, using **simplified** and repetitive **communication methods**. The caregiver needs to be patient, rephrase information, and use gentle, reassuring gestures. In these situations, the creation of clear, structured routines is essential to reduce patient anxiety and facilitate care. Caregivers must also be alert to signs of confusion or agitation, which may indicate unexpressed pain, discomfort or dehydration, and respond quickly and appropriately.

Preventing undernutrition is also a major challenge for frail, elderly patients. As we age, our nutritional needs change, and many patients suffer from loss of appetite, swallowing problems or dental difficulties that complicate their diet. Malnutrition can lead to loss of muscle mass, increase the risk of falls and weaken the immune system. It is therefore essential to offer balanced meals adapted to their specific needs, giving priority to foods that are easy to chew and swallow. The caregiver, by being present at mealtimes, must ensure that the patient is eating sufficiently, and report any changes in appetite or weight. Simple interventions, such as splitting meals into smaller portions or offering fortified foods, can make a big difference to the patient's overall health.

Elderly patients, especially those confined to bed or wheelchairs, are also at risk of **developing pressure sores**, which appear as a result of prolonged immobilization. Preventing these skin lesions is essential when caring for the frail elderly. Caregivers should **regularly change the** patient's **position**, use specialized cushions or mattresses to reduce pressure on certain areas of the body, and frequently check the condition of the skin. In the event of reddening or early signs of pressure sores, prompt action must be taken to prevent tissue deterioration.

Psychological support also plays a fundamental role in the care of elderly patients. Many elderly people suffer from social isolation, depression or anxiety, exacerbated by loss of autonomy and reduced social interaction. The caregiver, by virtue of his or her proximity to the patient, can play a central role by providing a sympathetic ear, engaging in regular conversation, and stimulating participation in adapted social or cognitive activities. These moments of interaction, however simple, are essential for improving patients' mood and quality of life.

Last but not least, it is vital to involve **families** in the care of frail, elderly patients. The family often plays a crucial role in supporting the patient, but they can also be faced with emotional difficulties, particularly in the face of their loved one's deteriorating state of health. The caregiver must not only accompany the patient, but also support the family, keeping them informed of health developments, answering their questions, and reassuring them about the care provided. Fostering open communication and involving relatives in certain care decisions creates a more serene, collaborative care environment.

The role of the caregiver in clinical trials
- Participate in the follow-up of patients included in research protocols

Participating in the **follow-up of patients included in research protocols** is an essential responsibility in the healthcare field. These protocols, also known as clinical trials, are rigorous studies conducted to evaluate the efficacy and safety of new treatments, drugs or medical interventions. The patients who take part play a key role in the advancement of medicine, and their follow-up requires special attention and increased vigilance on the part of caregivers. Taking part in this follow-up not only means ensuring that research protocols are rigorously applied, but also guaranteeing that patients benefit from human support throughout the study. This mission combines a scientific approach with careful attention to patients' physical and emotional needs.

One of the most important aspects of monitoring patients included in a research protocol is the **rigorous application of guidelines**. Clinical trials follow very strict protocols, designed to ensure the scientific validity of results while guaranteeing patient safety. Every intervention, medication or medical examination must be carried out in accordance with the rules established for the study. The caregiver, although often supporting the doctor or nurse in charge of the trial, must ensure that these steps are rigorously followed, whether in administering treatments or collecting the necessary data. This includes tasks such as monitoring vital signs, observing side effects and managing routine interventions, all the while remaining vigilant to the smallest details.

Constant vigilance is crucial to ensure patient safety throughout the trial. Patients participating in research protocols often receive experimental treatments, which may have unknown or poorly documented side-effects. Monitoring clinical signs is therefore fundamental to the early detection of any adverse effects or complications. Caregivers must be particularly attentive to subtle changes in the patient's condition: a variation in temperature, a change in vital parameters, or unusual symptoms must be immediately reported to the medical team. This careful monitoring not only ensures patient safety, but also provides valuable data for the research team on treatment efficacy and side effects.

In addition to clinical monitoring, psychological and human accompaniment of the patient is another central aspect of follow-up in a research protocol. Participating in a clinical trial can generate **worries** and **anxieties** in patients. The idea of receiving experimental treatment, often in a context where standard therapeutic options are limited, can be a source of stress. Patients may have doubts about the efficacy of the treatment, or fear potential side effects. The caregiver, by virtue of his or her proximity to the patient, plays a key role in providing moral support, answering questions and ensuring that the patient feels understood and cared for. Listening and empathy are essential to help the patient through this sometimes uncertain period.

Respect for informed consent is also a fundamental element of research protocols. Patients participating in these studies must be fully informed of the objectives of the trial, the treatments they will receive, the potential benefits, and the associated risks and uncertainties. If informed consent is initially collected by the physician, the caregiver must ensure that the patient continues to understand the various stages of the trial and what is expected of him or her. Furthermore, consent is an ongoing process: at any time, the patient must be able to ask questions or express concerns. The caregiver therefore plays the role of **mediator** between the patient and the research team, facilitating communication and ensuring that the patient's rights are always respected.

Another important aspect of patient monitoring in research protocols is **treatment management** and **error prevention**. Clinical trials often involve complex treatment regimens, with specific dosages, precise time windows for drug administration, and sometimes comparative treatments (placebo vs. active treatment). The caregiver must ensure that treatments are administered precisely, that doses are respected, and that administration schedules comply with the protocol. In addition, they may be involved in collecting data on patient **compliance**, i.e. ensuring that patients follow instructions correctly, that they take their treatment at home if necessary, and that they comply with study instructions.

Data collection is another essential aspect of patient follow-up in clinical trials. Every piece of data collected - whether clinical parameters, responses to treatment, or side effects - contributes directly to the evaluation of the efficacy of the experimental treatment. The caregiver may be responsible for collecting certain data, such as laboratory test results, quality of life questionnaires or clinical observations. This information must be rigorously collected and accurately documented, as it plays a key role in the final analysis of the trial. Any omission or error in data collection can compromise the scientific validity of the study, making rigor essential at every stage of the process.

The caregiver can also play an important role in the **practical management of** appointments and patient visits. Research protocols often require a very precise follow-up schedule, with regular visits for medical examinations, blood sampling, or monitoring the patient's progress. The caregiver can be involved in organizing and coordinating these visits, ensuring that the patient adheres to the trial schedule and is well informed of key upcoming dates. This ensures that the necessary data is collected at the right time, and that the patient's follow-up is continuous and protocol-compliant.

The **management of side effects** and serious adverse events is also a priority in the follow-up of patients included in clinical trials. If a patient develops side effects related to the experimental treatment, it is essential that these events are **immediately reported** to the research team for prompt and appropriate evaluation. The caregiver must be trained to recognize these effects, document them accurately and know when to alert the doctor in charge of the trial. This not only ensures patient safety, but also provides valuable information on the tolerability of the treatment being studied.

- ○ Medication management and specific care for patients in clinical research

Managing drugs and **specific care for patients in clinical research** is a complex and highly regulated task that demands absolute rigor from caregivers. Patients taking part in clinical trials often receive experimental treatments or drugs that are not yet available on the market. This calls for meticulous monitoring to ensure both patient safety and the scientific validity of the results. Every aspect, from drug administration to the management of side-effects, and the precise documentation of each stage, must be carried out with the utmost care.

One of the key aspects of drug management in clinical research is the **administration of experimental treatments** in strict compliance with the study protocol. Unlike standard treatments, clinical trials follow very specific guidelines, dictating when, how and at what dose drugs should be administered. The caregiver, often in collaboration with nurses and doctors, must ensure that each drug is administered according to the precise rules laid down by the protocol. This includes checking dosages, administration schedules and any special conditions associated with each drug, such as whether it should be taken on an empty stomach or after a meal, or whether it requires special monitoring after administration.

In addition to administering medication, the caregiver must also **monitor treatment compliance**. This means checking that the patient is complying with the prescribed treatment, especially when this includes a degree of self-management by the patient, such as taking tablets at home. In such cases, the caregiver may have to explain clearly to the patient how and when to take his or her medication, answer questions and ensure that instructions are understood. The caregiver must also gather information on the patient's **compliance**, i.e. whether he or she is scrupulously following the instructions for taking the medication, and whether he or she is not experiencing any difficulties in adhering to the protocol.

Another key aspect of medication management in clinical research is the **prevention of medication errors**. In clinical trials, these errors can have serious consequences not only for the patient's health, but also for the validity of the study results. Experimental drugs are often administered at very precise doses, and any error in dosage can distort the results of the trial. The caregiver must therefore adopt **strict verification procedures**, such as double-checking doses with another caregiver, or using traceability systems to ensure that the drugs administered correspond to the protocol prescriptions. They must also be alert to possible interactions with other treatments the patient may be taking, to avoid any interference that could affect the efficacy or safety of the experimental drug.

Monitoring side effects is also a central dimension of patient care in clinical research. Experimental drugs, by their very nature, can have unknown or unexpected side effects. It is therefore essential to set up continuous monitoring to rapidly detect any abnormalities in the patient's state of health. The caregiver, in his or her role as local contact, must be particularly attentive to subtle signs of side effects, such as variations in blood pressure, temperature, nausea, or changes in the patient's general condition. Every side effect, however minor, must be accurately documented and immediately reported to the research team, as this information is crucial in assessing the tolerance and safety of the treatment.

Clinical data collection associated with drug management is another crucial aspect. In a clinical trial, every intervention, every medication taken and every patient reaction must be carefully recorded in the study file. This data makes it possible to monitor the patient's progress, measure the efficacy of the treatment, and detect any potential problems. The caregiver may need to record data such as vital signs, symptoms reported by the patient, or the results of follow-up examinations. The accuracy of this documentation is essential to ensure that the trial results are scientifically valid and can be used to evaluate the treatment.

Clinical trials also often involve the use of **placebos**, which are administered to certain patients to compare the effects of the experimental drug with those of an inactive treatment. Although the caregiver is not informed of the division of patients into placebo and active groups (this information is often "blinded" to avoid bias), he or she must treat all patients in the same way. He or she must ensure that every patient receives the same level of care and monitoring, regardless of the treatment they are receiving. This maintains the integrity of the study while ensuring that every patient receives optimal care.

Managing interactions between treatments is also a sensitive issue. Patients included in clinical trials are often taking other medications for chronic or acute conditions, in addition to the experimental treatment. It is therefore crucial that the caregiver regularly checks concomitant treatments to ensure that they do not interfere with the research protocol. This includes checking for potential drug interactions, but also advising patients on what they can and cannot take alongside the experimental treatment (dietary supplements, herbal remedies, etc.).

Finally, it's important to stress that drug management in clinical trials also requires **fluid communication** with the patient. Patients may have doubts or concerns about an experimental treatment, and it is essential to reassure them, answer their questions, and make sure they understand the instructions. The caregiver must play a **mediating** role, facilitating communication between the patient and the research team, explaining procedures and ensuring that the patient feels supported throughout the trial.

Chapter 9

Therapeutic patient education in urology

The caregiver's role in patient education
- ○ Explain care and treatment to patients and their families

Explaining care and treatment to patients and their families is an essential task in the caregiver-patient relationship, which goes far beyond the simple transmission of medical information. It's about creating an environment of trust, where patients and their families feel supported, understood and involved in decisions concerning their health. The quality of this communication plays a decisive role in treatment adherence, anxiety management and overall patient well-being. Explaining care in a clear and appropriate way ensures that patients and their families understand what is at stake in the proposed treatments, their benefits and risks, and what each step entails. This promotes patient-centred care that respects the patient's needs.

The first step in explaining care is to **create an open, reassuring space for dialogue**. It's vital to ensure that the patient and family feel comfortable asking questions, and expressing concerns or doubts. The caregiver, often on the front line of care, must establish a relationship of trust based on listening. A calm environment and kind language help to reduce barriers and encourage more fluid communication. When patients and their families feel listened to and understood, they are more inclined to ask questions and express their concerns, enabling explanations to be tailored to their specific needs.

The **language used** in these exchanges should be simple, understandable and free of medical jargon. Even if certain medical notions are complex, it is possible to explain difficult concepts using simple words and analogies adapted to the patient's situation. For example, rather than talking about "venous thrombosis", a caregiver might say, "It's a clot that blocks the flow of blood in a vein, a bit like when a blockage forms in a water pipe." This approach makes the subject more accessible and less intimidating for patients and their families. It's also important to regularly check that the patient understands the information given, by asking questions or inviting them to rephrase what they've understood.

Another essential aspect is the **individualization of explanations**. Each patient is unique, and it is necessary to adapt explanations to his or her level of understanding, emotional state, and specific concerns. For example, an elderly patient with cognitive problems may need short, repeated explanations, while a young adult may seek more technical details for reassurance. The caregiver must be able to adapt to these different needs, taking into account the specificities of the patient and his or her family. In addition, some families may have cultural or religious beliefs that influence the way they perceive medical treatment. It is essential to listen to these concerns and adjust explanations to take account of these factors, in order to respect their values while explaining the benefits of the proposed care.

When it comes to complex or long-term treatments, such as chemotherapy, dialysis or palliative care, it's important to **break down information** into clear steps. It's often counterproductive to inundate patients and their families with technical information all at once, as this can overwhelm them and generate anxiety. It's best to start with the essentials, such as the treatment objectives, before moving on to the practical details of how it will be administered, the duration of treatment and possible side effects. This step-by-step approach **gradually** familiarizes patients and their families with the treatment process, answering their questions as they go along.

Another key element in explaining care is **managing expectations**. Patients and their families can sometimes have unrealistic expectations of treatment outcomes, hoping for a quick cure or the immediate disappearance of symptoms. It is essential to communicate clearly what treatments can offer, without raising false hopes. For example, in the case of a chronic disease such as diabetes, it may be necessary to explain that treatment will not cure the disease, but will help to manage it better and prevent long-term complications. It's also important to talk about possible

side effects, while reassuring patients that these are monitored and manageable in most cases.

Explanations of care and treatment also include **practical demonstrations** where necessary. For patients or families who have to manage home care, such as inserting a urinary catheter, administering insulin, or changing dressings, it's crucial to show them how to proceed, step by step. A practical demonstration followed by repetition of these gestures by the patient or his or her family will ensure that they feel confident to carry out these tasks once at home. The caregiver must ensure that these gestures are fully understood and mastered before leaving the patient or family to their own devices.

Finally, it is essential to address **the** issue of **patient autonomy and their role in care**. Encouraging patients to take responsibility for their own care, wherever possible, helps to reinforce their sense of control over their health and improve their adherence to treatment. This may involve advice on the adoption of healthy lifestyle habits, such as a suitable diet or physical activity, or education on the monitoring of certain parameters, such as blood sugar levels for a diabetic patient. By involving patients in the management of their own care, we give them the tools they need to better understand their disease and actively contribute to their own well-being.

Equally important is the **involvement of the family** in explaining care, as they are often a source of support for the patient. The caregiver must include relatives in these discussions, taking care to answer their questions and allay their fears. This enables the family to better understand the situation, provide adequate support to the patient and play an active role in monitoring treatment, especially in cases where the patient may have difficulty understanding or remembering information. The family thus becomes a key partner in the management of the patient's health, helping to ensure better continuity of care.

◦ Information on healthy living after surgery

Informing people about the lifestyle they should adopt after surgery is a crucial step in ensuring optimal recovery and preventing post-operative complications. After an operation, the body is in a convalescence phase where it needs adapted care, appropriate nutrition, sufficient rest and moderate physical activity to gradually regain its normal functions. The caregiver plays a key role in this process, explaining to the patient, and sometimes his or her family, the best practices to follow to support recovery. A healthy lifestyle after surgery not only facilitates healing, but also strengthens the immune system and minimizes the risk of infection or complications.

The **first recommendation** to convey to the patient concerns the importance of a **balanced diet**. After surgery, the body needs specific nutrients to regenerate. A diet rich in proteins, vitamins and minerals is essential for tissue repair and strengthening the immune system. For example, the proteins contained in meat, fish, eggs and legumes are essential for wound healing. It's also important to consume sufficient **vitamin C**, found in fruits such as citrus fruits, as it plays a key role in the production of collagen, a protein that helps tissue repair. Explaining this to patients can help them make dietary choices that promote faster healing.

Hydration is also a fundamental aspect. After an operation, it is common for patients to become dehydrated, particularly as a result of anesthesia, medication or bleeding. It is essential to encourage the patient to **drink enough water** throughout the day to promote blood circulation, maintain good kidney function and prevent constipation, a common side effect after surgery, especially if opioid analgesics are used. The caregiver must stress the importance of regular drinking, while adapting to the patient's specific needs, as in the case of certain procedures where water restrictions may be necessary, for example after kidney surgery.

Post-operative pain management is another aspect of healthy living after surgery. Pain, although common after surgery, must be well controlled to enable the patient to mobilize and gradually resume daily activities. The caregiver must explain to the patient the importance of **following analgesic prescriptions** without waiting for the pain to become too intense, as this can delay recovery. It is also important to reassure the patient that the pain will subside over time, and that non-medicinal techniques such as relaxation or the application of cold or hot compresses can also help relieve it.

Another crucial point in the information given to the patient concerns the **management of wounds and dressings**. After an operation, it is essential to keep the surgical wound clean and dry to avoid infection. The caregiver must explain in detail to the patient how to **care for his or her scar**, whether by following instructions for changing dressings, or avoiding certain activities that could compromise healing. For example, it is often advisable not to wet the wound for the first few days, and to avoid pulling on stitches by lifting heavy objects. If the patient has to manage his own dressings at home, the caregiver should show him the correct method for changing them, stressing the importance of **washing his hands** before and after each manipulation to minimize the risk of infection.

One of the most important aspects of healthy living after surgery is **progressive mobilization**. After surgery, staying in bed for too long can lead to complications such as **deep vein thrombosis**, bedsores and respiratory infections. It is therefore crucial to encourage the patient to get up and walk, even short distances, as soon as medically possible. The caregiver must reassure the patient that moderate physical activity, adapted to his or her condition, is beneficial to recovery. Indeed, movement helps stimulate blood circulation, improve respiratory function and prevent complications associated with immobility. In some cases, it may be necessary to recommend specific exercises, such as deep breathing exercises for patients who have undergone thoracic or abdominal surgery, to prevent pulmonary complications.

However, it's also important to emphasize the **balance between rest and activity**. While mobilization is essential, the body also needs rest to heal. It is therefore necessary to explain to patients that rest periods must be respected, and that they must not exhaust themselves by trying to resume their usual activities too quickly. **Quality sleep** is essential to support the healing process, enabling the body to regenerate and strengthen its immune defenses. The caregiver can give advice on how to promote good sleep, such as avoiding stimulants at the end of the day, or creating a calm environment conducive to rest.

Another important point to address is **infection prevention**. After an operation, the immune system can be weakened, making the patient more vulnerable to infection. The caregiver must therefore stress the importance of maintaining good **personal hygiene**, including regular hand-washing and avoiding contact with sick people, especially in the first few days after surgery. In some cases, specific precautions, such as wearing a mask or limiting visits, may be necessary to protect the patient. It's also vital to explain to the patient how to recognize signs of infection, such as fever, redness or discharge from the wound, and what to do if infection is suspected.

Finally, managing **emotions and stress** is an integral part of a healthy lifestyle after surgery. Even successful surgery can be a source of anxiety for the patient, particularly with regard to uncertainties about recovery, pain, or the evolution of his or her state of health. The caregiver must take the time to explain that stress can slow healing, and that it is important to adopt relaxation techniques, such as breathing exercises or regular moments of relaxation. In some cases, the caregiver can also refer the patient to psychological support services if necessary.

Helping patients to manage their own health
  ◦   Helping understand ongoing care (home catheterization, catheters, etc.)

Assisting in the understanding of continuing care, such as home catheterization, catheter management, or other medical devices, is an essential task for caregivers, which must be carried out with precision and clarity. Continuing care often involves medical devices used over the long term for patients with specific needs, such as urinary difficulties, kidney problems or other chronic conditions. The role of the caregiver is to accompany the patient and family in understanding this care, ensuring that they are comfortable with the use of these devices, their maintenance and monitoring. This support process is crucial to preventing complications, promoting autonomy and guaranteeing untroubled care at home.

The **first step** towards understanding continuous care is to explain in a clear and accessible way the **function of the device** used, whether it's a urinary catheter, a central venous catheter, or an ostomy. It is essential that the patient and family understand why the device has been fitted and how it contributes to improving the patient's health or quality of life. For example, in the case of home bladder catheterization, the caregiver should explain that the catheter is used to drain urine when the patient is unable to do so naturally, either because of obstruction or paralysis. Understanding this function helps to reduce the anxiety of the patient, who may initially be reluctant to the idea of having a permanent medical device.

Next, the caregiver must demonstrate **how to use** the device **correctly**, and how to ensure that it is working properly. For example, in the case of urinary catheterization, the caregiver can explain how to attach the catheter correctly, how to empty the collection bag, and how to check that the urine is draining normally without obstruction. It is essential that each step is detailed and repeated as many times as necessary, ensuring that the patient or caregiver fully understands what needs to be done. Practical demonstrations followed by the patient or family performing the gestures are often necessary to ensure that they feel comfortable and confident in managing the device.

Another important aspect is to **emphasize the** rigorous **hygiene rules** that must be observed to avoid infection, particularly in the case of catheters or probes. These medical devices involve direct access to the body's internal systems, making them particularly vulnerable to infection. The caregiver must therefore stress the importance of thorough hand-washing before and after each manipulation, as well as disinfecting equipment where necessary. For a catheter, for example, it's crucial to explain how to change dressings using sterile techniques, how to clean the catheter exit port, and when it's necessary to contact a healthcare professional if there are any signs of infection (redness, pain, discharge). These precautions help minimize the risk of infection, while reassuring the patient about his or her ability to manage the device at home.

One of the major challenges of continuing care is often the **management of potential complications**. The caregiver must therefore inform the patient and his or her family of the warning signs to watch out for, so that they can react quickly if a problem arises. In the case of urinary catheterization, these may include a decrease in urine flow, cloudy or foul-smelling urine, or bladder pain, which may indicate obstruction or infection. For a venous catheter, signs of local infection (redness, warmth, swelling) or signs of a more serious complication, such as embolism or thrombosis, should be known to the patient and family. The caregiver must therefore provide clear explanations of these symptoms, stressing the importance of **promptly contacting a healthcare professional** if these signs appear.

The **prevention of immobility-related problems** is also an important element to integrate into continuing care, especially for bedridden patients or those with reduced mobility. Devices such as urinary catheters can be an obstacle to mobility, and the patient may be reluctant to move for fear of pulling on or damaging the device. The caregiver must then explain how to mobilize the patient safely, adjusting the positioning of devices to allow a certain level of physical activity. For example, he or she may show how to reposition a urinary catheter to avoid tugging, or how to protect a catheter during movement. Encouraging mobility is crucial to preventing complications such as pressure sores or respiratory infections, and it also helps to improve patient morale by enabling them to retain a degree of independence.

It is also important to integrate **continuous care** into the patient's daily life, by adapting the explanations to his or her lifestyle. The caregiver can advise the patient on how to manage the device in various everyday situations, such as washing, dressing, or even leaving the house. For example, in the case of a patient with an ostomy, it is important to explain how to maintain the ostomy pouch, how to change it, and how to live with this equipment while maintaining a good quality of life. The caregiver can also offer advice on how to integrate this care into a daily routine that is not too restrictive for the patient.

Finally, the caregiver must offer **psychological support** to the patient, as adapting to ongoing care can be a source of stress and anxiety. The presence of a permanent medical device, such as a catheter or tube, can affect self-image and lead to worries about the future. The caregiver must therefore encourage open exchanges with the patient, inviting him or her to express fears and doubts. By answering questions sympathetically and providing reassurance about the day-to-day management of the device, the caregiver helps the patient to accept his or her new situation and regain a degree of serenity. If necessary, the caregiver can refer the patient to psychological support services or groups of patients with similar experiences, so that they can share their feelings and receive practical advice.

- Provide post-operative follow-up: manage appointments, monitor recovery

Post-operative follow-up is an essential step in the care process, designed to ensure that recovery from surgery takes place in the best possible conditions. Post-operative care includes managing medical appointments, monitoring healing, controlling symptoms, and supporting the patient's physical and psychological recovery. The caregiver plays a key role in this phase, ensuring that the patient complies with post-operative instructions, follows prescribed treatments, and is able to ask questions or express concerns. This vigilance helps to prevent complications and ensure that recovery proceeds without hindrance.

One of the first responsibilities of post-operative care is the **management of medical appointments**. After surgery, patients often need to see their surgeon, or other specialists, to assess the progress of their recovery, remove stitches, or adjust treatments as their condition evolves. The caregiver must ensure that the patient is aware of these appointments, and that the dates are respected. This means reminding them of the importance of these checks, even if the patient is feeling well. Each appointment is an opportunity to check on the progress of healing, to ensure that the patient is tolerating treatment well, and to intervene rapidly if there are any signs of complications. The caregiver can help coordinate these appointments, particularly for elderly or vulnerable patients who may find it difficult to organize their follow-up independently.

Monitoring physical healing, and in particular scarring, is another central dimension of post-operative care. The healing process must be closely monitored to detect any infections or local complications. The caregiver must ensure that the patient understands how to monitor the wound and change dressings if necessary. He or she should explain to the patient any warning signs, such as excessive redness, discharge, swelling or unusual pain, which could indicate an infection or healing problem. If in doubt, the caregiver should encourage the patient to seek prompt medical attention, as early intervention can prevent complications from worsening. In addition, it is often necessary to remind the patient of the hygiene instructions essential to healing, such as keeping the wound clean and dry, or avoiding certain movements to avoid pulling on the stitches.

Another important aspect of post-operative care is **pain management**. After surgery, it is common for the patient to experience post-operative pain, although this should diminish over time. It is essential to explain to the patient that pain can be controlled with prescribed medication, and that pain management is essential to enable progressive mobilization. The caregiver must also ensure that the patient takes his or her analgesics as prescribed, while making sure that he or she understands how to adjust the intake according to the evolution of the pain. If pain persists or worsens beyond what is expected, it is important to inform the medical team promptly, as this could indicate a complication.

Monitoring the patient's general condition after surgery is also crucial. Surgery, especially major surgery, can affect the whole body, and it is important to monitor the patient's vital signs and general condition in the days and weeks that follow. This includes monitoring temperature to detect infection, checking respiratory function, particularly if the patient has been under general anaesthetic, and assessing blood circulation, especially to prevent complications such as thrombosis. The caregiver should encourage the patient to remain attentive to his or her body and report any abnormal sensations, such as difficulty in breathing, swelling of the legs, or excessive fatigue, which may require medical intervention.

Progressive mobilization of the patient is another key element of post-operative care. After an operation, the risk of prolonged immobilization is a factor in complications such as bedsores and pulmonary embolisms. The caregiver must encourage the patient to mobilize as soon as possible, respecting medical instructions of course, and adjusting the activity according to the patient's abilities. This may involve taking a few steps in the room, then walking through the corridors of the hospital or home, depending on the patient's condition. Mobility promotes better blood circulation, speeds up muscle recovery, and helps improve the patient's morale. The caregiver must accompany this mobilization with care, taking care not to exceed the limits of the patient's capacity for effort.

Psychological support after surgery is just as important as physical follow-up. An operation, even a successful one, can be a source of stress and anxiety for the patient, particularly in the face of pain, uncertainties about recovery or the resumption of normal activities. The caregiver must listen to the patient's questions and concerns, reassuring him or her and providing appropriate answers. Sometimes, convalescence can seem long, and the patient may feel frustrated or discouraged. By offering moral support and encouraging regular exchanges, the caregiver helps the patient to maintain a positive frame of mind, and to look forward to recovery.

Informing patients and their families about ongoing care is also part of post-operative follow-up. In some cases, specific home care is required after discharge from hospital, such as changing dressings, managing a catheter, or taking scheduled medication. The caregiver must ensure that the patient and family fully understand this care, by showing them the correct actions to take and encouraging them to ask questions. It is often useful to provide written support or practical cards so that the patient and family have a reminder of the steps to follow when they return home. This helps to ensure that care is carried out properly, and reinforces the patient's autonomy in his or her care.

Finally, it is crucial to address the **prevention of long-term complications**. Some surgeries, such as orthopedic or cardiovascular procedures, require lifestyle adjustments to optimize recovery and prevent recurrence. The caregiver can advise the patient on aspects such as diet, smoking cessation, weight management, or the implementation of an adapted physical activity routine. By ensuring that the patient understands the importance of these preventive measures, the caregiver contributes to reducing the risk of future complications and improving the patient's long-term health.

Collaboration with nurses and doctors for therapeutic education

  ◦   Organize information sessions for patients

Organizing information sessions for patients is an essential part of helping them understand their condition, the treatments they receive, and the care they need to follow. These sessions play a key role in strengthening communication between caregivers and patients, increasing adherence to treatment, and helping them to better manage their disease. They enable complex information to be conveyed in a clear and accessible way, while offering patients a space to ask questions and express their concerns. Organizing such sessions requires careful preparation and a tailored approach to meet the varied needs of patients.

The first step in organizing a successful information session is to **clearly define the objectives**. It's essential to know what type of information needs to be communicated. Is it to explain a particular pathology, detail a specific treatment, or inform about the management of a medical device such as a catheter or stoma? Objectives should be centered on patients' needs, and each session should focus on information that is practical and directly applicable to their situation. For example, in a session for diabetic patients, the objective might be to teach them how to manage their blood sugar levels, understand the importance of nutrition, and know how to administer their insulin independently.

Secondly, it is crucial to adapt the **teaching method** to the patient's level of understanding. Not everyone has the same medical knowledge, nor the same comfort level with technical terms. It is therefore essential to choose **clear, simple language**, avoiding overly complex or jargonous terms. Explanations must be adapted to each type of audience, whether older adults, young adults or children, taking into account each person's ability to assimilate the information. The use of visual aids such as **slide shows, videos or illustrative diagrams** can be particularly useful in ensuring better comprehension. For example, to explain insulin treatment, showing a diagram of the pancreas and how insulin works in the body can help make concepts more tangible and concrete.

The **structure of the session** needs to be well thought out to ensure that information is conveyed progressively and in an accessible way. It's important to start the session with a **simple, clear introduction** to the subject, explaining the objectives of the meeting. Thereafter, it is useful to organize the information into logical, coherent steps. For example, in a session on post-operative pain management, it might be a good idea to start with an explanation of the causes of pain, before detailing the medicinal and non-medicinal options for managing it. A well-structured session makes it easy for patients to follow the reasoning and acquire the information in a fluid, progressive way.

A fundamental aspect of these **sessions** is to **encourage interactivity**. It's not just about imparting information, but also about creating a space where patients can ask questions and share their experiences. Information sessions should include **question-and-answer** sessions, where patients have the opportunity to ask for clarification on what they didn't understand, or to express personal concerns. The caregiver or healthcare professional leading the session should be an active listener, patient, and answer questions clearly and reassuringly. This not only helps to reinforce understanding of the information, but also helps to establish a climate of trust and safety for patients.

What's more, it's essential to **involve families and caregivers** in these sessions, as they often play a key role in the day-to-day management of the disease. By explaining care and treatment to loved ones, they can better support the patient, whether in managing treatment at home, organizing care, or keeping track of medical appointments. For example, in a session on caring for a patient after heart surgery, the family needs to understand the importance of monitoring certain warning signs, such as chest pain or shortness of breath. Involving family members in therapeutic education creates a stronger support system around the patient, increasing the chances of following recommendations and avoiding complications.

It is also important to **provide written materials** or take-home documents at the end of each session. These can summarize the key points of the session, reiterate essential instructions or offer practical tips on how to manage daily life with the disease. They serve as a reference for patients when they return home, helping them to apply the knowledge they have acquired. These materials should be written in simple language and illustrated where possible, so that they can be easily understood and consulted. For example, a guide to using a glucometer for a diabetic patient could include step-by-step instructions with illustrations for each phase.

The **frequency of information sessions** should also be adapted to patients' needs. For some, a single session may be sufficient to understand care or treatment, but for others, regular follow-ups may be necessary, especially if disease management is complex or progressive. For example, for patients with chronic illnesses such as kidney failure or cancer, regular sessions can help adjust information as their condition evolves or new treatment options become available.

Another point not to be overlooked is the importance of offering a **space for emotional support** during these sessions. Patients, especially those suffering from chronic or serious illnesses, may experience anxiety or stress in the face of treatment. These information sessions provide an opportunity to address these emotional aspects and offer psychological support. The caregiver can, for example, reassure the patient that it's normal to feel overwhelmed at first, and that over time, managing care will become more familiar and less stressful. Additional resources, such as support groups or patient associations, can also be offered, so that participants can exchange ideas with others going through similar experiences.

Finally, it's important to **solicit feedback** from patients at the end of the sessions. Asking their opinion on the clarity of the information provided, on the aspects they found most useful, or on points that could be improved, enables future sessions to be tailored to their actual needs. This guarantees continuous improvement of the sessions, and ensures that the content remains relevant and effective for each patient group.

◦   Adapt speech to patients' level of understanding

Adapting speech to the patient's level of understanding is a fundamental skill for any caregiver. Every patient has different cognitive abilities, medical knowledge and experiences, which means that the same message cannot be communicated uniformly to everyone. The aim is to ensure that every patient, whatever their education or condition, fully understands the care and treatment they are being offered. Not only is this essential for good medical care, but it also helps to build patient confidence, encourage adherence to treatment and reduce anxiety.

The first step in adapting your speech is to **assess the patient's level of understanding**. This can be done by asking simple questions about their knowledge of their own illness or treatment. For example, in the case of a diabetic patient, the caregiver may ask what he or she knows about managing blood sugar levels, or about the foods he or she can eat. This approach gauges the patient's starting point, without making them feel uncomfortable or judgmental. Another way of assessing understanding is to observe the patient's reaction during the explanations: if he or she seems confused or asks a lot of additional questions, this may indicate that he or she needs more explanation or simplified language.

Once the level of understanding has been assessed, it is essential to **simplify the language used**. Medical terms are often complex and technical, and can easily confuse patients who are unfamiliar with medical vocabulary. It is therefore important to translate these terms into simple, understandable words. For example, instead of "venous thrombosis", we can say "blood clot" and explain that it blocks the flow of blood through the veins. Using everyday terms makes it easier to understand, and helps patients to better grasp their illness or treatment. It's also a good idea to check regularly that patients are following the explanations correctly, by asking them to rephrase what they've understood.

Using **metaphors or analogies** is another effective way of helping patients understand complex concepts. Comparing the human body to something more familiar can greatly enhance understanding. For example, to explain how arteries clogged with cholesterol plaque work, we can use the analogy of water pipes clogged with limescale, explaining that the flow of water (or blood) becomes more difficult when there is a blockage. These mental images facilitate understanding by linking abstract concepts to more concrete, familiar experiences for the patient.

In addition to simplified language, it's crucial to adapt **the amount of information** provided. Some patients may feel overwhelmed if they are given too much information at once, especially after the announcement of an illness or before surgery. In such cases, it's important to **balance the explanations**, introducing the most essential concepts first, before moving on to more complex details. For example, for a patient about to undergo surgery, it may be more reassuring to begin by explaining the aims of the operation and the expected benefits, before going on to detail the technical aspects of the procedure. Dividing the explanations into stages helps to make the information more digestible, and prevents the patient from feeling lost or anxious.

Another important aspect is to ensure that **information is repeated and re-explained** if necessary. Some patients, especially when stressed or tired, may have difficulty retaining information. So don't hesitate to rephrase explanations several times, using different words or concrete examples. In addition, it is often useful to offer **written or visual aids** to complement oral explanations. These aids enable the patient to reread and assimilate the information at his or her own pace, once back at home. For example, an illustrated guide to managing diabetes, with simple images and step-by-step instructions, can be a valuable tool to help a patient better understand how to measure blood sugar levels or adjust his or her diet.

It's also essential to **adapt your speech to the patient's emotional state**. When a patient is anxious, frightened or upset by a diagnosis, their ability to understand and assimilate information may be impaired. In these situations, it's important to adopt a reassuring tone, show empathy and take the time needed to answer all their questions. It's often helpful to break down information and not overload patients with too many details, especially when they're in a state of shock. For example, after a cancer diagnosis, the caregiver may focus first on emotional support and immediate practical information, such as the first stages of treatment, before returning later to the technical details of treatment options.

Involving the **family or close friends** can also help to adapt the message. Some patients, particularly the elderly or frail, may find it difficult to assimilate information on their own. Involving a loved one in discussions ensures that someone else understands the instructions, and can support the patient in managing his or her care at home. What's more, family members can ask additional questions that the patient might not dare to ask themselves, or clarify points that the patient may not have understood. This ensures better continuity of care and follow-up after the consultation.

Finally, to make sure that the speech is well adapted to the patient, it's important to **ask for feedback**. Encouraging the patient to express what he or she has understood, or what remains unclear, enables the caregiver to readjust his or her discourse in real time. It also helps to establish a dynamic in which the patient feels comfortable asking questions and actively participating in managing his or her own health. For example, after explaining a drug treatment, the caregiver may ask the patient: "Does this seem clear to you? Is there anything you'd like me to clarify?" This shows the patient that his or her questions and doubts are legitimate, and that the caregiver is there to help him or her understand, without judgment.

Conclusion: The future of the orderly in urology

Future challenges for urology care
- An aging population and an increase in urological pathologies

The **aging of the population** is a global phenomenon with major repercussions on the healthcare system, particularly in the field of urology. With increasing life expectancy, more and more people are reaching an advanced age, and this aging is accompanied by a significant increase in **urological pathologies**. These conditions, which mainly affect the urinary system and male reproductive organs, are becoming increasingly common as the population ages. Urology, as a medical specialty, must adapt to this reality, as diseases such as prostate disorders, urinary incontinence and kidney failure affect a growing number of elderly people, requiring specific and often prolonged care.

One of the most common urological pathologies in the elderly is **benign prostatic hyperplasia (BPH)**, an enlargement of the prostate gland. This condition, which affects almost all men over the age of 50, can lead to urinary difficulties, such as a frequent urge to urinate, low urine stream pressure, or a feeling of incomplete bladder emptying. Although benign, BPH can significantly affect men's quality of life, disrupting their sleep and limiting their daily activities. As the population ages, this condition is becoming increasingly common, and urology departments are having to adapt their care to meet the needs of an ageing population. Treatment can be medical or, in some cases, surgical, and often requires regular follow-up to monitor disease progression.

Prostate cancer is another urological pathology directly linked to age. It is the most common cancer in men, and its incidence increases with age, mainly affecting men over 65. While some prostate cancers progress slowly and simply require active surveillance, others can be more aggressive and require rapid management, with treatments ranging from surgery to radiotherapy or hormone therapy. As the population ages, more and more cases are diagnosed each year, posing challenges in terms of early detection and appropriate treatment. The challenge for caregivers is to offer an individualized approach, taking into account the patient's biological age, other comorbidities and quality-of-life preferences.

Urinary incontinence, another common disorder among the elderly, affects both men and women. With age, the muscles of the pelvic floor and bladder lose their tone, which can lead to involuntary urine leakage, particularly during physical exertion, coughing or sneezing (stress incontinence). This condition is not only physically embarrassing, but can also have a significant psychological impact, causing embarrassment, shame and sometimes **social isolation**. The aging of the population is considerably increasing the prevalence of this pathology, forcing healthcare professionals to adapt management strategies. These strategies range from perineal re-education to medical treatment, including devices such as catheters or absorbent pads, and sometimes surgery.

In addition to prostate problems and incontinence, aging is associated with an **increased risk of urinary tract infections**. In the elderly, urinary tract infections such as cystitis are common due to a number of factors. Age-related decline in immune function, urinary retention due to pathologies such as BPH, and the use of medical devices such as urinary catheters all increase the risk of infection. These infections can lead to serious complications, including urinary sepsis, and must be treated promptly. UTIs in the elderly can also cause atypical symptoms, such as confusional states, making diagnosis more difficult. Prevention, including adequate hydration and regular monitoring, is essential to reduce the occurrence of these infections.

Chronic renal failure is another urological pathology commonly associated with aging. Kidney function naturally declines with age, and in some people this decline may be accelerated by chronic diseases such as hypertension or diabetes, both of which also increase with age. Kidney failure can progress slowly and without symptoms until it reaches an advanced stage, making regular check-ups crucial for the elderly. When kidney function is severely impaired, treatments such as dialysis or kidney transplantation may be necessary, although these options are not always feasible or desired by older patients, due to their general frailty. The management of renal failure in the elderly therefore requires a multidisciplinary approach, taking into account not only renal function, but also the patient's general state of health and quality of life.

The **aging of the population** also poses specific challenges for urological palliative care. Many urological pathologies in the elderly, such as advanced cancer or end-stage renal failure, require end-of-life care that must be tailored to each patient's individual needs. Palliative care aims to relieve pain and other symptoms, while offering emotional and psychological support to patients and their families. The role of the care team is to offer care that focuses on quality of life, taking into account patients' wishes regarding their end of life, while ensuring that treatments are in line with their needs and values.

Finally, the ageing of the population means that **healthcare services** need to be rethought to cope with the increase in urological pathologies. Caregivers not only need to be trained in the specificities of urological care in the elderly, they also need to have the appropriate resources to offer effective management. Prevention and early detection are essential to minimize complications, but this requires infrastructures capable of handling the growing demand. In addition, with the increase in chronic pathologies, it becomes crucial to develop strategies to optimize home care and reduce hospitalization, by offering older patients long-term follow-up solutions.

        ◦   Developments in care techniques and robotization
The **evolution of care techniques** and the rise of **robotization** in the medical field mark a major turning point in the way patients are cared for and treated. These technological advances have transformed medical practices, improving the precision of interventions, reducing risks for patients and optimizing care

processes. While technology continues to advance at a steady pace, it offers new possibilities for more effective, less invasive care that is better adapted to individual needs. However, these innovations also pose challenges, particularly in terms of training, accessibility and the relationship between caregiver and patient.

One of the most significant advances in medical care is the **introduction of surgical robotics**. Since the first robot-assisted interventions, this technology has developed rapidly to become an indispensable tool in certain disciplines, notably urology, cardiac and orthopedic surgery. The **Da Vinci robot**, for example, is one of the most widely used systems in hospitals worldwide. It enables surgeons to perform complex procedures with **enhanced precision** and **3D visualization**. Thanks to its extremely precise articulated arms, this robot offers greater freedom of movement than the human hand, and reduces the surgeon's natural tremor. This means that delicate operations, such as prostatectomy or kidney surgery, can be performed far less invasively than with traditional techniques. Patients benefit from **smaller incisions**, **reduced bleeding**, **less post-operative pain** and **shorter recovery times**.

In addition to robotics, the **development of minimally invasive surgical techniques** has radically transformed the way operations are performed. Laparoscopic surgery, which involves operating through small incisions using a camera and fine instruments, has become a common alternative to open surgery. This technique not only reduces scarring and the risk of complications, but also shortens hospital stays. For patients, these advances mean a better post-operative experience and a faster return to normal life. Combined with robotization, robot-assisted laparoscopy represents a further step towards increasingly sophisticated care that is less traumatic for the body.

Artificial intelligence (AI) is also playing a growing role in the evolution of healthcare techniques. It is used to **analyze massive quantities of medical data**, helping with diagnosis, therapeutic decision-making, and even the prediction of treatment outcomes.

For example, in the field of medical imaging, AI algorithms can analyze scans or MRIs to detect anomalies, such as tumors, faster and sometimes more accurately than the human eye. This enables **earlier detection** and **more targeted interventions**. In oncology, AI is used to personalize treatments according to a patient's genetic profile, optimizing the chances of success. In hospitals, too, AI is helping to **optimize resource management**, by scheduling appointments, managing patient flows or tracking drug stocks.

In the field of **rehabilitation and physiotherapy**, robotization has also brought major innovations. **Exoskeletons** are now used to help patients regain mobility after accidents or surgery. These devices, which support the body's limbs while facilitating movement, enable patients to **relearn to walk** or regain the use of their limbs with robotic support. Rehabilitation robots are programmed to adapt to the patient's progress, increasing or decreasing assistance as required. This technology opens up new prospects for patients suffering from partial or total paralysis, promoting faster, more effective recovery.

Technological advances are not limited to surgery and rehabilitation. In the field of **nursing**, robotization is also beginning to play an important role, notably with the emergence of **assistance robots** that help nursing staff with daily tasks. These robots can transport medication, move bedridden patients or perform surveillance rounds. By freeing up time for nursing staff, these technologies enable nurses and orderlies to concentrate more on human care, such as listening to patients and providing them with psychological support. Robotization in this field helps to **optimize hospital management** and **reduce physical fatigue** among caregivers, while guaranteeing rigorous monitoring of logistical tasks.

Alongside robotization, the **development of remote monitoring technologies** is also revolutionizing the management of chronic patients and post-operative follow-up. Thanks to connected devices such as sensors or smartwatches, it is now possible to monitor patients' vital signs at home. This includes monitoring blood pressure, heart rate, oxygen levels or blood sugar levels. These data are then transmitted in real time to doctors, who can intervene rapidly in the event of any anomaly. This means **fewer hospital admissions** and more **proactive management of** patients, especially those suffering from chronic illnesses such as diabetes or heart failure. Care thus becomes more personalized, with continuous monitoring that improves patients' quality of life while optimizing the use of medical resources.

However, the rise of robotization and new technologies in healthcare also poses **challenges**. First of all, there's the question of **training**. Caregivers, whether doctors, nurses or care assistants, need to acquire new skills to use these technologies safely and effectively. Training to handle surgical robots, for example, requires specific and rigorous training. What's more, healthcare professionals need to be able to work collaboratively with AI systems, while retaining their clinical judgment and their central role in the patient relationship.

The other challenge is **accessibility**. While robotization and advanced technologies offer cutting-edge care, they are often costly and not always accessible in all healthcare establishments, particularly in rural areas or developing countries. It is therefore essential to find solutions to democratize these technologies, so that they benefit as many people as possible and do not further exacerbate inequalities in access to care.

Finally, the question of the **caregiver-patient relationship** remains crucial. Although robotization and AI are improving the efficiency and precision of care, it's important to preserve the humanity in care. Technologies must not replace human interaction, but rather support it, enabling caregivers to devote more time to listening, empathizing and accompanying patients.

The growing role of the caregiver in a changing medical context

   ∘   Towards greater responsibility in care

The trend towards **greater responsibility in care** marks a profound change in the way patients participate in the management of their own health. In the past, the caregiver-patient relationship was based on a hierarchical dynamic in which the patient was often passive, relying on decisions made by healthcare professionals. Today, thanks to changes in attitudes, technologies and medical practices, patients are increasingly encouraged to play an active role in their care. This increased empowerment is based on the idea that patients, as actors in their own health, are better placed to make informed decisions, manage their day-to-day well-being and proactively prevent complications.

The first lever of this growing sense of responsibility is **access to information**. The Internet and new technologies have profoundly changed access to medical knowledge. Patients can now search for information on their illnesses, treatments and available care options. This **democratization of medical information** enables individuals to better understand their state of health and ask more pertinent questions of their doctor. However, one of the challenges is to ensure that patients have access to reliable and validated information, as the mass of online information is often difficult to sort through. This is why healthcare professionals have an essential role to play in guiding patients to credible sources of information, and helping them to interpret this data appropriately.

This empowerment also requires more open and collaborative **communication between caregiver and patient**. Medical decisions are no longer solely in the hands of caregivers. Today, medicine is moving towards an increasingly **partnership-based** approach, in which the patient is involved in every stage of the care process. This means empowering patients to participate in the decisions that concern them, whether it's the choice of treatment, pain management or the planning of an intervention. Caregivers need to be able to explain the available options clearly and support the patient in making informed decisions. This builds trust between patient and caregiver, while encouraging patients to take an active part in their own recovery or disease management.

Another key aspect of this increased sense of responsibility **is therapeutic education**. It's not enough for patients to be informed about their disease; they must also be trained to manage their condition on a daily basis. Therapeutic education aims to give patients the skills they need to monitor their health, adjust their treatments if necessary, and prevent complications. For example, for a diabetic patient, this means learning how to measure blood sugar levels, adapt their diet and administer insulin according to their needs. This empowerment enables patients to take better control of their health, reduce their dependence on the healthcare system and avoid avoidable hospitalization.

Connected technologies, such as **remote monitoring devices**, have also fostered this empowerment. Connected objects, such as smartwatches, blood pressure monitors or glucose meters, enable patients to track their health parameters in real time and transmit this information to their medical team. This continuous monitoring helps patients **anticipate health problems** before they become critical. For example, a heart patient can monitor his or her heart rhythm and detect abnormalities before a crisis occurs. By empowering patients to manage their day-to-day health, these technologies encourage a more proactive approach and help prevent many complications.

Accountability in care is not limited to chronic disease management. It also plays a crucial role in **prevention**. By empowering people to take responsibility for their lifestyles - diet, physical activity, alcohol and tobacco consumption - caregivers help them become aware of their role in maintaining their health. Prevention and education campaigns on risky behaviours aim to make people aware of the importance of their daily choices. For example, the fight against smoking or the promotion of physical exercise are designed to make people aware of their responsibilities, and to make them realize that they have a direct influence on their future health. By raising awareness of risks and protective behaviours, we encourage people to take responsibility for their own health, and to take steps to preserve their well-being.

Medication management is another area where empowerment plays a major role. More and more, patients are being encouraged to understand the importance of their treatment and to follow it rigorously. Adherence is a key factor in ensuring the effectiveness of treatments, particularly for chronic diseases. Patients must not only understand why they are taking a medication, but also be aware of the consequences of poor compliance. In the case of hypertension, for example, failure to take medication correctly can lead to serious complications such as stroke. By reinforcing this sense of responsibility, caregivers aim to reduce the risk of non-adherence and improve therapeutic outcomes.

However, this increased empowerment comes with its own **challenges**. Not all patients have the same capacity to appropriate information or manage their health independently. Elderly people, for example, may need extra support to understand and apply medical recommendations, particularly in managing connected devices or monitoring health parameters. Similarly, people with low levels of health literacy may find it difficult to navigate medical information and understand the issues involved in their treatment. In such cases, it is essential that caregivers adapt their approach to meet the specific needs of each patient, taking into account their level of understanding and social context.

Finally, patient responsibility for care must always be **balanced** with constant support from caregivers. It is important not to transfer the entire responsibility for health onto patients' shoulders, as this could generate pressure or anxiety. Empowerment should be seen as a **partnership** between the patient and the care team, where the patient is encouraged to play an active role, but can count on the support and guidance of healthcare professionals to accompany them throughout their care journey.

◦ Helping patients to manage their own health

Supporting patients in the self-management of their health is a key process in the evolution of modern medical care. Self-management, which is based on the idea that patients take an active part in managing their own well-being, does not mean that the caregiver removes himself or herself from the equation. On the contrary, it's a partnership in which caregivers provide patients with the knowledge, tools and support they need to manage their health independently and effectively. This model not only improves patients' quality of life, but also boosts their self-confidence, while reducing dependence on constant medical care.

Self-care begins with **thorough therapeutic education**. Patients need to understand their illness, its symptoms, the risks involved and what they can do to prevent complications. To achieve this, the caregiver or healthcare professional must be able to **explain medical information in a** way that makes it accessible and understandable. For example, for a patient suffering from diabetes, it's not enough to tell them to monitor their blood sugar levels; it's essential to explain why this is important, how fluctuations in blood sugar levels affect their body, and what concrete actions they can take to regulate it on a daily basis. The aim is to help patients integrate this knowledge into their routine in a fluid, autonomous way.

One of the first elements of self-management is **taking charge of daily treatments**. Whether for chronic diseases such as diabetes or hypertension, or for conditions requiring regular care, patients must learn to manage their treatments rigorously. This involves knowing when and how to take medication, but also recognizing possible side effects and adjusting dosage according to medical instructions. To this end, the caregiver plays a **guiding** role, checking that the patient understands the instructions and proposing solutions for integrating these treatments into daily life. For example, the use of pillboxes, telephone alarms or applications to monitor medication intake can facilitate this management. If patients are well informed and monitored, they become more comfortable managing their treatment independently, knowing that they can consult their caregiver in case of doubt or difficulty.

Another essential aspect of self-management support is **lifestyle adaptation**. Many chronic pathologies require changes to lifestyle habits, whether in terms of diet, physical activity or stress management. Caregivers have a fundamental role to play in supporting and monitoring these changes. Let's take the example of a hypertensive patient: it's crucial that he understands the importance of reducing his salt intake, increasing his fruit and vegetable intake, and adopting regular physical activity. But beyond providing information, the caregiver needs to help the patient **put** these changes **into practice**, by suggesting achievable and realistic goals. This could involve setting small challenges, such as replacing salty snacks with fruit, or walking for 30 minutes a day. These changes, while accessible, can have a major impact on disease management.

In this context, it is also essential to address the **monitoring of health parameters**. Thanks to technological advances, patients can now monitor several aspects of their health themselves at home, such as blood pressure, blood sugar levels or oxygen saturation. The caregiver must train the patient to use these devices and, above all, to **read and interpret the results**. It is important to ensure that the patient knows how to recognize normal values and those that should alert him or her. For example, a diabetic patient needs to be able to take his or her blood sugar and understand whether it's within a normal range, or whether he or she needs to adjust treatment or consult a doctor. This gives patients greater autonomy, while encouraging them to remain vigilant about their health.

Support for self-management is not limited to the physical aspect, but also encompasses the **emotional management of** the disease. Living with a chronic illness or managing regular treatments can be a source of anxiety, frustration and discouragement. The caregiver must not only meet physical needs, but also offer psychological support. For example, helping a patient to better manage stress through relaxation techniques, breathing exercises or the integration of a meditation routine can be beneficial. Encouraging patients to **share their emotions**, whether with loved ones or in support groups, is also an important aspect of this support. By listening to patients' concerns and encouraging them to verbalize their difficulties, caregivers can help them come to terms with their situation and develop coping mechanisms to help them live better with their illness.

Self-care also means knowing when to **ask for help**. It is essential to remind the patient that being autonomous does not mean managing everything alone. The role of the caregiver is to instill the necessary confidence in the patient to know when to consult a healthcare professional, especially in cases of doubt or unusual symptoms. For example, a patient suffering from heart failure needs to know how to recognize the warning signs of an exacerbation, such as increased breathlessness or swollen ankles, and understand that in these situations it is necessary to contact a doctor immediately.

Finally, support for self-management must be **gradual**. Not all patients have the same adaptability or confidence to manage their health independently. It is therefore essential to tailor support to each individual's abilities and pace. For some, it will be possible to quickly delegate much of the health management, while others will need ongoing support and regular monitoring to feel comfortable. It is crucial that the caregiver is flexible and adjusts his or her interventions according to the patient's progress, while maintaining a constant dialogue to ensure that the patient feels supported on his or her journey.

Training to progress in the nursing auxiliary profession
   ◦   Access to specializations
Specialization in the healthcare field is an essential pathway for healthcare professionals wishing to broaden their skills, acquire

cutting-edge expertise and meet the increasingly complex needs of patients. Specializing not only enables them to develop in-depth expertise in a specific medical discipline, but also to embark on a dynamic process of personal and professional development. In a context of rapidly advancing technological, scientific and therapeutic progress, specialization has become an essential lever for improving the quality of care, while opening up new career prospects for caregivers.

The first step towards a specialization is often motivated by **the desire to deepen a knowledge or passion for a particular field**. Whether it's oncology, pediatrics, geriatrics, cardiology or urology, each specialization offers the opportunity to explore a medical discipline in depth and acquire specific skills that will enable them to better respond to the clinical challenges encountered by patients. For a healthcare professional, the decision to specialize is also an opportunity to focus on pathologies, treatments or types of care that require particular expertise. For example, a nurse specializing in intensive care acquires unique skills in caring for critically ill patients, while an orderly trained in gerontology can offer optimal support to the frail elderly.

Becoming a specialist requires **in-depth, ongoing training**. In many healthcare systems, this involves specialized training programs, certifications, practical internships and, often, a final exam to validate the skills acquired. Caregivers can thus follow specific curricula that will enable them to master the theoretical and practical aspects of their specialty. This training, which can last several months or years depending on the specialty, combines both academic courses and periods of practice in a clinical environment, under the supervision of experienced professionals. For example, for a healthcare professional wishing to specialize in **medical resuscitation**, training will include familiarization with the state-of-the-art equipment used in intensive care, learning complex protocols, as well as hospital internships to gain essential practical experience.

One of the defining aspects of the specialization pathway is the importance of **mentoring and hands-on learning**. Beyond academic knowledge, specialization involves a progressive immersion in the practice of care, where caregivers learn from seasoned professionals. This mentoring process is fundamental, as it enables the acquisition of subtle skills that are difficult to teach in a theoretical setting alone. By observing, asking questions and taking an active part in care on a specialized ward, trainee nurses can refine their gestures, develop their capacity for clinical analysis and learn to manage crisis situations or complex cases. In disciplines such as neonatology, where every gesture must be precise and measured, experiential learning is essential to develop the necessary dexterity and responsiveness.

Specialization also opens the door to **new career opportunities**. Specialized caregivers are highly sought after in hospital departments, specialized care centers, private clinics or rehabilitation facilities. Expertise in a particular field allows you to stand out on the job market and choose more targeted, better-paid positions. What's more, in some healthcare systems, specialization can offer opportunities for advancement in the professional hierarchy, enabling a caregiver to take on greater responsibility or become a benchmark in his or her field. For example, a nurse specializing in **anaesthesia** may not only be able to work in operating theatres, but also play a key role in post-operative pain management and critical care.

Specialization also enables us to **meet the changing needs of the population**. With an aging population, an increase in chronic diseases and technological advances in care, medical specialties are called upon to diversify and adapt. Caregivers need to be able to cope with complex situations and pathologies that are more frequent in ageing populations, such as neurodegenerative diseases and cancer. For example, a specialization in **oncology** enables a caregiver to learn about the latest treatments, such as immunotherapy or targeted therapy, and to offer holistic support to patients throughout their journey, from diagnosis to palliative care.

One of the major challenges in accessing specialization is **continuing education**. In a field as dynamic as healthcare, knowledge evolves rapidly, and new techniques and protocols appear regularly. As a result, specialized caregivers need to engage in a continuous training process, to keep abreast of advances in their discipline. This can take the form of attending **medical congresses**, seminars, online training courses, or reading scientific articles. For example, a carer specializing in **cardiology** will need to keep abreast of new treatments for heart failure, or advances in minimally invasive cardiac surgery. This capacity for continuous learning is essential to guarantee quality care and remain competitive in a constantly evolving field.

Finally, specialization does not mean confining oneself to a narrow field, but rather **broadening one's horizons** by collaborating with other medical specialties. Modern healthcare is increasingly based on a multidisciplinary approach, where specialists from different fields work together to provide comprehensive, coordinated care for patients. A urology specialist, for example, frequently collaborates with oncologists, radiologists and nutritionists to develop individualized treatment plans for prostate cancer patients. This interdisciplinary collaboration not only enriches the skills of the caregiver, but also enhances the quality of care and ensures comprehensive, personalized management.

o   Career prospects in the urology department

Career prospects in the urology department are vast and varied, offering healthcare professionals many opportunities to evolve, specialize, and contribute to ever-changing areas of care. Urology, which deals with disorders of the urinary system in men and women, as well as disorders of the male genital organs, is a key medical specialty. It encompasses fields as diverse as the treatment of urinary tract infections, urological oncology, prostate surgery, incontinence management and kidney transplantation. For doctors, nurses and care assistants, working in this sector offers opportunities for advancement and specialization in response to the challenges posed by an aging population and an increase in chronic diseases.

For **doctors**, career prospects in urology are particularly promising. After studying general medicine, future urologists undergo specialized training, often accompanied by a period of hospital residency, during which they acquire practical expertise in the various facets of urology. A urologist's career can then evolve into various sub-specialties, depending on interests and patient needs. For example, a doctor may choose to specialize in **urological oncology**, a rapidly expanding field due to the prevalence of prostate cancer and kidney tumors. This choice enables them to work on cutting-edge treatments, such as robotic surgery or immunotherapy, in partnership with other specialists like oncologists and radiotherapists.

Urologists can also move into the fields of **reconstructive surgery** or **renal transplantation**, two specialties that combine advanced surgical skills with multidisciplinary patient management. Kidney transplantation, for example, requires close collaboration with nephrologists, immunologists and intensive care teams to ensure successful surgery and long-term follow-up of transplanted patients. This specialization enables us not only to intervene in critical situations, but also to restore a significant quality of life to patients suffering from end-stage renal failure.

For **urology nurses**, the career prospects are just as attractive. Nurses play a central role in the care of urology patients, whether in hospital, outpatient or home care settings. Their role extends far beyond basic care, as they are often responsible for **therapeutic education**, helping patients to understand their treatment, manage medical devices such as urinary catheters, and recognize signs of complications. Nurses may also specialize in specific areas such as **incontinence management**, working with patients suffering from post-surgical or age-related urinary disorders, particularly in geriatric wards.

By specializing, nurses can acquire highly specific **technical skills**, such as assisting with complex urological surgeries or managing post-operative care in minimally invasive surgery units. The development of robotic surgery in urology, for example, has opened up new opportunities for specialist nurses, who are now trained to work closely with surgeons during these high-precision procedures. Nurses can also become involved in **palliative care teams**, where they play a crucial role in accompanying patients with advanced urological cancers, providing pain control and psychological support.

For **nursing assistants**, the urology department also offers interesting prospects, particularly in terms of day-to-day patient care. Often working in close collaboration with nurses and doctors, care assistants are responsible for many aspects of basic care, but their role is not limited to that. In a urology department, they are actively involved in **monitoring patients after surgery**, managing urinary catheters, and educating patients about home care, particularly in the case of chronic pathologies. Their work demands constant vigilance, particularly in preventing infections, monitoring wounds and assisting patients with their daily routine.

The professional development of nursing assistants can also involve further training, enabling them to **specialize in certain types of care**, such as the management of invasive medical devices or palliative care in urology. In addition, care assistants can become **urology referents** within their department, enabling them to coordinate care, supervise new caregivers, and improve day-to-day practices. This specialization gives them invaluable expertise, which may lead them to take on greater responsibilities, particularly in terms of team coordination.

Beyond purely clinical prospects, the field of urology also offers career opportunities in **research** and **teaching**. Constant advances in the treatment of urological pathologies, such as new robotic surgery techniques or advances in immunotherapy for prostate cancer, require healthcare professionals trained in clinical research. Working in urology research means being at the forefront of medical innovation, contributing to the development of new treatments and participating in clinical trials. Urologists, nurses and other specialized healthcare professionals can also play an essential role in teaching, passing on their knowledge and skills to new generations of caregivers through continuing education programs or in medical and nursing schools.

At the same time, **careers** in **health management** and **administration** are also options for experienced urology professionals. With the growing need for specialized care and an aging population, the management of urological services is becoming a major challenge for hospitals and clinics. Healthcare professionals who have acquired solid clinical expertise can progress to positions in coordination, department management or healthcare project management, playing a key role in optimizing resources and improving the quality of care offered.

www.ingramcontent.com/pod-product-compliance
Lightning Source LLC
Chambersburg PA
CBHW072148290526
45794CB00004B/1446